# VICTOR BONNEY

*The Gynaecological
Surgeon of the Twentieth Century*

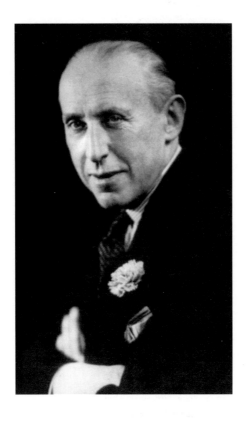

# VICTOR BONNEY

## The Gynaecological Surgeon of the Twentieth Century

### Geoffrey Chamberlain

RD, MD, FRCS, FRCOG, FACOG(Hon), FFFP(Hon)

Emeritus Professor of the University of London
St. George's Hospital, London, UK

with a foreword by

### Professor Robert Shaw

President, Royal College of Obstetricians and Gynaecologists
London, UK

## The Parthenon Publishing Group

International Publishers in Medicine, Science & Technology

NEW YORK                                    LONDON

Published in the USA by
The Parthenon Publishing Group Inc.
One Blue Hill Plaza, PO Box 1564, Pearl River
New York 10965, USA

Published in the UK and Europe by
The Parthenon Publishing Group Ltd.
Casterton Hall, Carnforth, Lancs., LA6 2LA, UK

**Library of Congress Cataloging-in-Publication Data**
Chamberlain, Geoffrey, 1930–
    Victor Bonney : the gynaecological surgeon of the twentieth century /
Geoffrey Chamberlain ; with a foreword by Robert Shaw.
        p. ; cm.
    Includes bibliographic references and index.
    ISBN 1-85070-712-X (alk. paper)
    1. Bonney, Victor, 1872–1953. 2. Gynecologists--England--Biography. 3.
Surgeons--England--Biography. 4. Generative organs--Surgery--England--
History--20th century. I. Title
    [DNLM: 1. Bonney, Victor, 1872–1953. 2. Gynecology--England--
Biography. 3. Gynecologic Surgical Procedures--history--England. WZ 100
B7175C 2000]
    RG76.B66 C48 2000
    618.1'0092--dc21
    [B]                                                    00-056683

**British Library Cataloguing in Publication Data**
Chamberlain, Geoffrey, 1930–
    Victor Bonney : the gynaecological surgeon of the twentieth century
    1.Bonney, Victor 2. Gynecologists - Great Britain - Biography 3. Surgeons -
Great Britain - Biography
    I.Title
    618.1'45'092

    ISBN 1-85070-712-X

Printed and bound by Bookcraft (Bath) Ltd., Midsomer Norton, UK

# CONTENTS

There can be no doubt that Victor Bonney was recognised as a leading, if not the foremost, gynaecologist of the first half of the twentieth century. His reputation was worldwide, extending not only throughout the then British Commonwealth of Nations but within Europe and the United States of America – a reputation founded not only on his gynaecological surgical skills, but on his innovations in surgery and his teaching abilities.

In partnership with Sir Comyns Berkeley, his more senior colleague for many years at the Chelsea Hospital for Women and the Middlesex Hospital, he demonstrated the value of radical abdominal hysterectomy for cancer of the cervix. Their results would be viewed as exceptional, but when one considers the absence of antibiotics, blood transfusion and modern anaesthesia, the outcomes must be viewed as even more spectacular and indicative of the quality and immense surgical skills of the operators. Whilst extended gynaecological surgery techniques for malignancies were important developments, so too were the contributions from Bonney in developing conservative gynaecological surgical procedures – particularly those of ovarian cystectomy and, of course, myomectomy. It is the latter technique with which Bonney's name is so intimately connected, both in terms of results and recorded follow-up data, and also with the development of specific instrumentation – many examples of which are still used today and have not been bettered.

His publications and writings were also extensive. The publication of the textbook *Gynaecological Surgery* (jointly with Sir Comyns Berkeley), first in 1911, and on to a fourth edition in 1942, was always associated with highly complimentary reviews, and it rapidly became established as the standard text of the era. The text had a uniquely personalised presentation and contained numerous unique illustrations of operative procedures.

Bonney was a stalwart supporter of the Royal College of Surgeons throughout his career and being a gynaecologist, with no real clinical interest in obstetrics, was not supportive of the development of the British College of Obstetricians and Gynaecologists founded in 1929. This, I believe, reflected his then belief in the need to maintain gynaecology within the broader sphere of surgery as a whole. He was elected Senior Vice-President of the Royal College of Surgeons in 1937 and indeed left a bequest as well as many papers and documents to that College. It is perhaps with some irony that the College for which Bonney did so much work should have since cast away the opportunity of continuing to commemorate one of its greatest Vice-Presidents, while the College against whose formation he argued now continues that commemoration through the annual award of our prestigious Victor Bonney Lectureship.

Professor Robert Shaw
President, Royal College of Obstetricians and Gynaecologists

V ictor Bonney was a primary influence on world gynaecology in the years between the wars. He led by example, being a greater surgeon than many; his teaching actively passed on his ideas to his juniors who in turn left the imprint on their pupils. Thus a third generation of gynaecologists are still using the best of Bonney's techniques some 50 years after his death. His attitudes had been formed in the Victorian and Edwardian times. Perhaps a little rigid in outlook, Bonney's attitudes mirrored those of the poet Rudyard Kipling whom he greatly admired, and so I have used appropriate extracts from Kipling's poems to head each Chapter.

As acknowledged elsewhere, many helped me write this book but notably George and Peggy Bonney, his surviving family. The pleasure of seeking out information from a previous era has been enormous and has opened this contemporary surgeon's eyes to the problems of his predecessors.

Geoffrey Chamberlain
Emeritus Professor of Obstetrics and Gynaecology
St. George's Hospital, London

## ABOUT THE AUTHOR

Geoffrey Chamberlain is a retired Emeritus Professor of Obstetrics and Gynaecology from the University of London. Like Victor Bonney, he was a consultant obstetrician at Queen Charlotte's Hospital and a consultant gynaecologist at Chelsea Hospital for Women in his earlier career, becoming Professor at St. George's Hospital Medical School in the latter part of his professional life. He has written many textbooks and lectured widely on his subjects but this is his first non-technical book.

Professor Chamberlain lives in Gower, South Wales with his wife, also a medical professor, and their short attention-spanned Dalmatian. There, in his retirement, he is an active member of the History of Medicine Department at the Welsh School of Medicine in Cardiff.

N o book about history could be written by one man without the help of many others. The family of George Bonney, Victor Bonney's nephew and heir, have been most helpful in allowing me access to the material that Bonney left in his home and in providing accounts of his later days. I have spent many hours in their company and have enjoyed all of them. Bonney's handwritten account of his life is in 50 exercise books, which provided me with many of his opinions. I am most grateful to many gynaecologists who have told me of the professional times they spent with Bonney, particularly to John Howkins, Leonard Easton and Bancroft Livingston who helped me with material for this book. Barry Jackson (President of the Royal College of Surgeons of England), Robert Shaw (President of the Royal College of Obstetricians and Gynaecologists), Tom Lewis, John Malvern and Martin Quinn have also been helpful in providing extra material.

The literature of Bonney's life and work is enormous and I would like to thank the librarians and archivists of the Royal College of Surgeons, the Royal College of Obstetricians and Gynaecologists and the Middlesex Hospital Medical School. I am most grateful also to the librarians who collected material and helped me at the Welsh School of Medicine, the London Metropolitan Archives and the Royal Society of Medicine.

Short quotations from the poems of Rudyard Kipling, which appear at the beginning of each chapter, have been reproduced with the kind permission of A P Watt Ltd (London).

I am most grateful to David Bloomer, managing director and publisher of the Parthenon Publishing Group, for having the courage to go outside his usual field and take on a biography, and to the staff of Parthenon for their careful work on the manuscript.

My wife very kindly read through the manuscript spotting any errors, while Sally Lyne read the manuscript and gave me a non-medical view of the content. My secretary, Caron McColl, worked hard at this book dealing with drafts and rewrites and I am most grateful to her for her patience and intelligent collation of my words and writing. Any remaining mistakes are my own.

GVPC

*'The years, as they roll by, leave behind them memories which increasingly pile up until, when 80 years have tolled, they form a large untidy heap which, if sorted out, would be the history of a life.'*

From a speech prepared by Victor Bonney in 1952 for his eightieth birthday dinner. This had to be postponed because of his illness, and sadly never took place.

# CHAPTER ONE

# CHILDHOOD
## *1872–1890*

*If you can fill the unforgiving minute*
*With sixty seconds' worth of distance run*
RUDYARD KIPLING, *IF*

Victor Bonney was born at three o'clock in the morning of December 17, 1872 at the family home at 320 King's Road, Chelsea, which looked down on Poulton Square. The boy was named William Francis Victor Bonney, the first names being after his maternal and paternal grandfathers, respectively. In later life Bonney would slightly resent these extra names, but it was the tradition then to involve as many of the parents and grandparents in the child's name as possible. In his earliest scientific papers, published from 1903, Bonney signed himself as William Francis Victor Bonney, but by 1906 this had contracted to Victor Bonney and he used the initials VB for his artist's work. So it remained for the rest of his life.

Victor was the eldest child, with brothers Jack and Ernest Henry following in 1874 and 1875. Whilst Victor appeared to have a healthy infancy, Jack was feeble and fed on 'scientific feeding stuffs', the details of which we do not know. William Bonney (Figure 1), Victor's father, was a general practitioner in Chelsea, as had been his father before him. The Bonneys were of French origin, being descended from the de Bonney family, who were originally from Burgundy, with branches in Champagne and Lorraine.

It was from this last group, who came to Britain with the Huguenots, that Victor's own stock derived. His mother, Anna-Maria, was a Poulain, one of the French aristocratic families who stayed in France throughout the French Revolution. She was descended from the de Graimbergs, who moved to Heidelberg after the Revolution, changing their name to von Graimberg (Figure 2).

Victor was born in politically restive days. Gladstone was at the zenith of his power as Prime Minister. His radical government aimed to abolish class privilege and determined to provide a wider cross-

1

section of society with political, economic and cultural opportunities. His cabinet led the abolition of political patronage for public office, requiring instead an open competitive examination for entry to the civil service. The educated classes were achieving more influence over the declining hereditary aristocracy. A *cause célèbre* had been the Education Act two years before Bonney's birth, a major tool of emancipation providing free, almost universal primary education. At its very heart, however, lay ammunition for Gladstone's Nonconformist detractors; it eventually sowed the seeds of his defeat by the Tories under Disraeli in 1874.

Victor was brought up in a medical family. His grandfather, Dr Francis Bonney, practised in Brentford, Middlesex; he died when Victor was five. His father, Dr William Bonney, was 32 when Victor was born and had qualified from the Middlesex Hospital in 1863. He started his Chelsea practice in 1869 and worked there for 50 years. He was a man of strong opinions and attitudes, an attribute that he passed to Victor. William Bonney kept a lifelong interest in medicine and was renowned for his natural powers of storing up, and profiting by, his past clinical experiences with patients.

There was a red lamp posted over the front door of the family home on the King's Road, as was common for doctors' houses in the late nineteenth century. Telephones were unusual, and if a doctor was required, a messenger or relative would call at the doctor's house requesting a house visit or sometimes requesting a bottle of medicine, which would be wrapped up in shiny white paper, carefully creased and folded, and a red wax seal added on the top. Usually a shilling was charged for advice and a bottle of medicine. As the nineteenth century passed, the consulting room of the surgeon apothecary was 'no longer exposed to the vulgar gaze' and the magnificent glass globular flasks of coloured liquids were removed from the front windows of the house to those of the pharmacist. Bonney recalled his father's practice later:

'The drugs at the service of the physician remained much as they had been for the past 100 years; mostly of vegetable origin with a few inorganic compounds thrown in. I used to help in my father's surgery long before I came to the Hospital, and even today the rows of labelled bottles in a dispensary have a fascination for me. Synthetic drugs were practically unknown; I think salicylic acid was the first of them, and I remember very well the appearance of antipyrin during the great influenza epidemic of 1891.' [1]

Victor's father had pneumonia in 1878 and afterwards travelled to Southsea to convalesce. This was used by the family as a reason for a holiday, with five-year-old Victor visiting the Royal Navy dockyard in Portsmouth, seeing for the first time HMS *Victory*, Lord Nelson's flagship at Trafalgar in 1805, by then preserved in her original state in a dry dock.

The house in Chelsea had a large back garden (Figure 3), large enough for a model train to run in it. The Bonney family had many artistic friends – painters and musicians – and their home was renowned for many years for the regular singing parties held there. Bonney thought then and later that singers should always accompany themselves at piano or lyre and did not think much of those who had to have a pianist to help set the note. Furthermore, he had strong views that, when performing, singers should always stand well and in a relaxed way.

When Victor was eight (Figure 4), the family moved to 145 Upper Beaufort Street on the west side of the Fulham Road. Like most small boys, his youthful passion was for food; he would later recall the plentiful bakeries and patisseries in that area. At that time, however, there was an absence of tea or coffee shops. For liquid refreshment, one had to visit a public house. In 1880, the ABC (Aerated Bread Company) opened its first shop, preceding Lyon's popular tearooms (1907) in providing clean, inexpensive food and beverages for large numbers of middle-class families. Its many tea shops lasted in London until well after the Second World War.

The town in which Victor grew up was very different from today. Thick 'pea-souper' fogs were common, and in winter the pavements and roadways were filthy with mud, horse droppings and straw, for horse-drawn carriages were the only means of transport. When someone was ill in the houses of middle-class Chelsea, straw was laid in the street to muffle the noise of horses and wheels. Crossing sweepers kept clear channels at intervals for pedestrians to cross the dirty road. Much tugging of forelocks and doffing of caps used to earn a halfpenny tip – woe betide the non-tipper for he would find himself accidentally sprayed with wet mud. Traffic jams were common. Horses reared in their tack and walking, even on the pavements, was hazardous. The horse buses rivalled each other to pick up passengers, often racing madly toward a potential traveller. At night, above the pandemonium, gas lights gave off a mellow yellow light. Victor would walk with his boots and gaiters getting dirty, but happy with the confusion.

William Bonney had a profound contempt for and dislike of schoolmasters, and so Victor was not at first sent to a regular school, his parents teaching him at home. When he was nine years old he went to Miss Parker's day school in Gunter Grove. In later years he would say that he could not remember what he learned there; his abiding memory was of perpetual war with the boys from the Clockhouse Board School, who used to make up a gang to bully the boys from the private school. Many routes home were used in order to avoid these clashes.

That year (1882) Bonney recalled that he went to see HMS *President* in the West India Dock. The successor to this ship became the base for the Royal Naval Volunteer Reserve, and later the Royal Naval Reserve, and was moored for many years on the Thames near the Middle Temple. She is now in private ownership there.

In 1883, when Victor was 11, his father was diagnosed as having aortic regurgitation. This did not mean a lot to a boy at the time, but Bonney had already noticed that his father had what he considered to be beautiful hands, which used to show palpitations in the 'large thin Filbert nails which were exceptionally big with well marked half moons'. His father also had mild diabetes, a condition which had been recently described but for which there was no treatment until Frederick Banting and Charles Best isolated insulin approximately 40 years later.

At the age of 12, Victor transferred to St. Mark's School in Fulham Road near Stamford Bridge. His father had not realised the importance of small boys mixing with others of the same age, and Victor had so far had an adult-oriented childhood. There were always enjoyable and social people calling at the family home, and Victor had many affectionate friends, but this was reflected in his dealings with his own age group. At school he was thought to be a little conceited and even to have a superiority complex. It was not until quite late in adolescence that he made friends of his own age.

Victor had quite broad knowledge and a quick-working brain at this stage; it was obvious that he enjoyed school. He used to wear Eton jackets and stiff collars, and would, like all small boys, complain about the amount of his homework. None of this stopped his development of an immense interest and joy in billiards, a game that was popular in the middle classes at this time; snooker had not been invented. This interest lasted throughout his life. Bonney had a billiard table in most of his homes later and he considered himself a very good player. He always thought it possible that had he not gone into medicine and instead been further trained in billiards, he could have turned professional.

At school a teacher named Mr Baggaley was well remembered by Bonney for imbuing him with an interest in Shakespeare. This lasted into later life, when Shakespeare was joined as a literary hero by the great English poet, Rudyard Kipling.

Victor was much attached to his mother, Anna-Maria, whom he admired enormously; by this time she led a quiet life as the matriarch of her family. As well as his brothers, the other companion of this rather solitary boy was Totty, a pug dog who was part of the family for some years. Victor was to become an adolescent with a cocky assertiveness, although he sometimes felt physically inferior for he was rather short.

Victor liked drawing and had a fine understanding of shape and perspective. His subjects were mechanical things such as ships and bridges rather than flowers or natural beauties that had more gentle curves. This gift persisted into adult life, both in his professional drawings of operations and his landscape watercolours. He also had a fine boy's soprano voice and would join in all the musical activities at home. It was from this age that Victor started mouth breathing. He attributed this to damage he had received to his nose in a childhood accident with a lamp post, but at about this time he took up boxing; this may have caused some damage to his nasal passages.

A great adventure for Victor in this year (1886) was being taken to see his adult friend Robert Stanley drill in the Volunteers' Manoeuvres on Wimbledon Common. These manoeuvres were an excuse for much local festivity and relaxed behaviour. Bonney remembered well the August days when the windmill at Wimbledon Common was surrounded by troops. The military would be camped out in tents; drill competitions and shooting matches would take place between the various regiments. Heavy artillery was fortunately forbidden because of the proximity of the houses on the periphery of the Common. It was a shooting accident a little after this time when a stray bullet ricocheted too far and landed in civilian property that caused the manoeuvres to leave Wimbledon. They went to Bisley, where the National Rifle Championships became the natural successor of the manoeuvres and are still contested between the services and civilian marksmen.

Victor used to sail his boat on the Round Pond in Kensington Gardens and described the great space between the Albert

Memorial (completed in 1876) and the Natural History Museum, where he would walk with his nanny or other members of the family up to the Gardens (the Science Museum and the extended Imperial College had yet to come). Bonney recalled children's dances of that time and, since his previous contact with females had only been his mother and her visiting friends, remembered vividly his heart being broken for the first time by a girl.

In 1887 came the Golden Jubilee of the ageing Queen Victoria. She had been on the throne since 1837, but after the death of her beloved Albert in 1862 had become a virtual recluse, rarely appearing in public. She kept a close interest in government affairs but complained bitterly at the volume of reading matter which Parliament and the Cabinet produced. She was the first monarch regularly to receive her Prime Ministers – Disraeli or Gladstone – who invariably had to travel to Balmoral, the Royal Family's Scottish Highland retreat, as the Queen spent much of her time there. However, given the national feeling, the Golden Jubilee could not be ignored and Queen Victoria arrived in London to ride in triumph in an open carriage whilst the country shouted its relief. Street parties were held and Queen Victoria retired back into her northern redoubt. She was to live on for another 14 years.

At the time of the Golden Jubilee, Britain was living in the Victorian sunset, exporting manufactured goods worldwide and receiving resources in return. Britannia was the leading colonial power, and the political map of the world was covered with pink areas to indicate the spread of her Empire. A major war had not been lost since Napoleonic times; there was a Pyrrhic victory against the Russians and victories against the Indians and the Sudanese. None of these were what could be termed military powers at the time, but the Victorian British considered their army to be invincible, a happy delusion that lasted until the end of the nineteenth century. The Zulus, and later a handful of Boer farmers in South Africa, demonstrated that they could take on the British army and upset the military order; 'we had no end of a lesson' (Kipling). Victor was brought up at the end of the Victorian era and many of his ongoing attitudes were created and moulded in this atmosphere.

In 1887, by now in a man's coat with a tall collar, Victor took the Cambridge local examination and passed with first class honours. The London matriculation was passed easily and in 1890 he made preparations for beginning a career in medicine.

# CHAPTER TWO

# MEDICAL APPRENTICESHIP
## *1891–1899*

*If you can dream – and not make dreams your master;*
*If you can think – and not make thoughts your aim*
RUDYARD KIPLING, *IF*

V ictor Bonney had naturally been influenced by the careers
of his father and grandfather and always wanted to go into
medicine; it had been his aim from his early teens. He was torn
between studying at St. Bartholomew's Hospital and the Middlesex
Hospital. In those days medical training was thought to be best at
the London medical schools, the few in the rest of the country being
perceived as provincial. He had visited the Middlesex and was very
impressed with the large wards with their observation windows at
the end, but he disliked what he thought was the persistent system
of patronage of medical staff which lowered its prestige. Bonney's
first choice was St. Bartholomew's and he records that he started
there in 1891 at the age of 18 under Thomas Horder (later Lord
Horder who cared for George V) to study biology, physics and chemistry, the old first MB course.

    'I travelled from and back to Chelsea by the river, on which there
ran a regular service of steamboats, a very pleasant means of transport. My alternatives were the old two-horse bus or the stuffy
Underground Railway, or my flat feet. Though there was a restaurant in the School, only relative plutocrats could lunch there and
most of us went to an ABC shop looking out on Smithfield and situated where the Pathological Block now stands. For fivepence you
could get there a cup of tea or coffee, a roll and butter and a slice of
cake, and it was extensively patronised by the more indigent students, of whom I was one, for my pocket money was only 5s. a week
and even then I was a heavy smoker. A favourite amusement was
throwing lumps of sugar (think of it in these days!) from the win-

dows of the upper room in which we fed at the drivers of passing vans and I remember one infuriated vanman raising Cain after someone had hit him fair and square on the cheek.' [1]

The story goes that Bonney left St. Bartholomew's hastily under a cloud, for he wrote almost perfect answers in the first examination. Bonney vehemently denied any misdemeanour, claiming that his excellent answers to the written questions were due to his near-perfect photographic memory.

'I must confess that I was a lazy and foolish student when at Bart's, and indeed for some years afterwards. Unfortunately I had a very good memory and could learn very quickly – what the actors call "a quick study". This gift, when conjoined with an immature mind, is a fatal one, for it promotes laziness and gives the ass something to be conceited about. The age at which individuals pass from adolescence into manhood is variable. I have known lads of 16 who for balanced outlook and resolute purpose were already fully grown men, and others who retained their larval form till well into the twenties. I was one of these latter.' [1]

Be that as it may, Bonney took the preliminary scientific examination for the Middlesex Hospital in biology, physics and chemistry, promptly failing in physics and chemistry. He resat them and passed easily. Hence, both medical schools can claim a hand in the early premedical training of Victor Bonney.

'And so in the autumn of 1891 I left [St. Bartholomew's] and went to Middlesex, but I had been long enough at Bart's to have become imbued with that reverence and affection which the fine old place inspires in all who work within its walls, and I felt keenly humiliated to leave it for a hospital so very much smaller and lacking its tremendous traditions. Looking back, however, I realise that the change was a fortunate one for me, since it led to me coming under the influence of a most remarkable man – John Bland Sutton – to whose inspiration is owing whatsoever I have succeeded in doing.' [1]

The Middlesex at this time was rising to the forefront of success, with staff including doctors serving the royal households, presidents of Royal Colleges and obstetricians such as William Duncan and Robert Boxal. Bonney's arrival at the bottom of the ladder at the

Middlesex was not marked with any great ceremony. He studied anatomy using his father's old second-hand books (but then anatomy had not changed much in the 30 years since William Bonney had qualified). Grey of St. George's Hospital had produced the popular anatomical volume that taught Bonney the basics of his anatomy. He remembered using a physiology book by Kirks, but anatomy was his first academic love.

Bonney still lived at home while he was studying at the Middlesex Hospital Medical School. The family moved in 1893 to 110 Elm Park Gardens on the east side of the road, a much larger house where the billiard table could have its place of honour. It was here that Bonney had his 21st birthday party. He was presented with a gold watch by his father; he very proudly kept this for the rest of his life. His scholastic career progressed, and Bonney took the London second MB in preclinical subjects in 1894. He reckoned that a short spell of intensive work just before examinations would save many wasted days of learning in a more systematic fashion. Bonney was not a good student, but enjoyed the arts and music. He wore the traditional frock coat and silk hat (as did many medical students at that time), buying a buttonhole each day for twopence. He continued this floral habit to the end of his adult life.

It was at about this time that Bonney's love of opera started, and he bought tickets to see such operatic luminaries as Jean de Reszke and Dame Nellie Melba. De Reszke was a Polish tenor who had a voice described as 'of exceptional beauty which he coloured with great skill'. His phrasing was impeccable while his personal charm made him one of the most popular artists of his time. He visited Covent Garden every year from 1887, singing parts as varied as Romeo and Tristan. The great Nellie Melba was an Australian soprano who appeared every season in London from 1889 to 1914, continuing again after the First World War. Starting as a high coloratura, her voice kept its freshness for many years and her brilliant techniques were amazing. She was *prima donna assoluta* who ruled the opera world for many years, and she later became one of Bonney's patients. Bonney was also most impressed by Francesco Tamagno, a tenor who became very popular in England and who had started singing the year Bonney was born. By 1890 he was considered the greatest *tenor di forza* in the world. It is said he had an extraordinary voice, and his upper range was such that he often found it easier to sing some arias a semitone or even a tone higher than they were scored. Bonney considered that Tamagno's voice was one of the purest he had heard and aimed at this standard himself. His boy's soprano was now past; it had matured to a fine tenor voice, which would now be considered to be almost a baritone in range. Bonney chose tenor parts for they were of far greater quality and range, and included considerably more opportunity for the singer to shine.

As Bonney moved on to his clinical years at the Middlesex, he began walking the wards, the classical Victorian tradition where young trainee medical students were assigned to be apprentices of the seniors, learning by their example. He was a dresser in the surgical wards and a clerk in the medical ones, but did little theoretical work. His early obstetrics was taught to him by his father, for midwifery could then be learnt out of the hospital in the local area under the tuition of a general practitioner. Deliveries took place in the Battersea slums, which were filthy and infested with parasites and vermin. Bonney learnt how to perform forceps deliveries and internal version of the baby there, kneeling on the floor in order to get a better angle of action. The neighbourhood was notorious, but doctors and their medical students walked freely and easily amongst the people, granted immunity from the less law-abiding citizens by virtue of their black Gladstone bags.

Bonney claimed at this time that he left for work without eating breakfast most days because he was late, ate no lunch because he was too poor, but went home for afternoon tea at about four o'clock, attending no late afternoon lectures.

Bonney's surgical studies were on the firm of Mr Hulke and he recalls the massive use of iodoform, a pungent antiseptic still used. Hulke was President of the Royal College of Surgeons and also President of the Geological Society, but died prematurely. Medical training as a student was mostly by practice and by watching one's seniors in the wards, the outpatient departments and the operating theatres. Contact with the honorary surgeons and physicians was tenuous. The firms of students and training doctors used to meet the honorary consultant at half past one in front of the hospital (in what is now the hospital's car park) and then escort them in to their wards or operating theatres.

'If the day was fine we would watch the honorary staff arriving in their carriage and pair. You must not think we were on intimate, or even on bowing terms with these great figures. There was an abyss, seemingly impassable, between them and us across which we looked with a veneration verging on idolatry.' [1]

Bonney did not like theoretical learning, but made reference in his journals to his use of Taylor's *Textbook of Medicine*, Walsham's *Surgery* and Galabins's *Obstetrics* as sources of reference. Most of the students' teaching was from the house surgeons or registrars who dealt with practical medicine. Ward rounds with them went on for many hours.

In July 1895, Bonney took the final qualifying examination of the Conjoint Board of the Royal Colleges of Surgeons of England and Physicians of London. He failed, but accepted this, for he had done no work. He revised intensively throughout the later summer months, benefiting from it as his memory was good. Although the books were teaching him a significant amount, he did little practical work because there were few patients available to him. Bonney passed obstetrics and surgery this time, but failed in medicine, where he had written a good paper but had done a poor clinical examination.

This was a watershed in Bonney's life; at last he realised that he should start working hard if he wanted to become a good doctor. From this point on he began to consider everything logically, so that rather than remembering isolated facts, he looked for trends to link information together. The following year he passed medicine with a distinction in the Conjoint Board examination and went on in the autumn to take the London third MB, which again he passed with distinction. This was a much stiffer examination than the Conjoint Board examination and carried more prestige. Despite his continued and dedicated revision timetable, Bonney also found time to go to hear Dame Clara Butt, the young contralto, who sang rarely at the opera, mostly keeping to the concert platform. Bonney tried to attend her concerts as often as possible.

Bonney became house physician to the great Douglas Powell, the Royal Physician, and to Sir Kingston Falker KCMG, KCVO. There was so much competition even for these types of house jobs that to obtain this post he had to take an examination. He was appointed, but soon fell foul of both his chiefs. He said that he made two major errors whilst working with this team of powerful doctors: the first was that he often treated the patients before his superior had seen them – this, in the field of internal medicine in the 1890s, was a terrible *faux pas*. The other error was that his notes were too brief, containing only the relevant facts. His superiors did not approve of this and he was heavily criticised for it. Additionally, his superiors were unhappy about Bonney's popularity as a teacher of students, amongst whom he was much sought after for his approach, which was both clear and precise.

After this first house physician's post he became a casualty officer at the Middlesex Hospital at the princely rate of £10 12s a quarter (80p a week now). Whilst that went much further in 1897 than now, it was still a comparative pittance. This was the year of Queen Victoria's Diamond Jubilee, an event that marked the end of a socially secure century and the birth of social revolution in Britain. Bonney's life was devoted to a debutante, May du Pasquier, the daughter of a family friend who lived in Charlton, to the southeast of London. Bonney would call upon her and walk home from there in the evening. It is not certain how deeply they became attached; Bonney considered they had a verbal engagement, but there was no reference to a ring, and he was saddened when he received a letter from her ending the relationship.

In January 1899, Bonney left the Middlesex Hospital and applied for the post of house physician at the Brompton Hospital. In this he was unsuccessful; he attributed this to the opposition of his two previous physician superiors who had never approved of his rather brisk and efficient manner of dealing with their patients at the Middlesex. Bonney had shown that he had little time for sitting around thinking about things in the contemplative way that general physicians were prone to do. He became a general practitioner locum in the Caledonian Road, since there were no vacancies at the Middlesex in internal medicine. He reapplied for a medical post in the Middlesex, but again was not supported. At this point he decided not to go any further with internal medicine and turned to a more active speciality. He took his primary examination for the Fellowship of the Royal College of Surgeons of England at six months' notice and, he later said of it, was fortunate in getting a question in the paper that referred to some work on appendicitis that he knew well, and therefore obtained a good pass.

A chance meeting with the most eminent surgeon and gynaecologist John Bland Sutton (later knighted) in the corridor of the Middlesex led to Bonney taking up a career in gynaecology. On hearing of his persistent lack of success in applying for medical appointments, Bland Sutton, with all the scorn he could muster, said, 'Nonsense, we want a house surgeon at the Chelsea; the job is vacant and I will see that you get it if you apply'. If this really occurred as related much later by William Gilliat in the Council of the Royal College of Obstetricians and Gynaecologists (RCOG) in 1953, we must be eternally grateful to the Middlesex for not appointing Bonney to the internal medicine staff.

Thus, at the end of June in 1899, Bonney came for the first time to Chelsea Hospital, where he started what was to become his life's work: gynaecological surgery.

'It was a mere chance which put me into Gynaecology; an accidental meeting in the corridor of the old Middlesex Hospital; for up to that moment I had planned to become a consulting physician, the subtle problems of medicine having a great attraction for me; and up to the present time, in spite of what the Communists would call my "deviation", my interest in them remains strong.'

Bonney entered into gynaecology, staying there all his professional life. He left the care of women the richer for his work.

# CHAPTER THREE

# GYNAECOLOGICAL TRAINING
## *1899–1905*

*If you can trust yourself when all men doubt you,*
*But make allowance for their doubting too*
RUDYARD KIPLING, *IF*

T he year before Victor Bonney was born, the Chelsea
Hospital for Women had been established at 178 King's Road
to treat 'women suffering from diseases especial to their sex'.
Around this time, general hospitals were loath to take women with
gynaecological problems as inpatients for little active treatment was
used in gynaecology and so most became long-stay patients – up to
10–12 weeks. James Aveling started his new hospital for 'gentle-
women of limited means and women of respectability'. He had come
to London from Sheffield, and some said that his motivation was
that he was too old to accept a junior position and yet not old
enough to obtain a senior appointment at an established London
hospital. The women admitted to the Chelsea Hospital for Women
were not the usual group to be given charity, but owing to the nature
of gynaecological conditions, it was felt they deserved a place of
their own. Aveling opened an outpatient clinic in the King's Road
and was soon joined by Robert Barnes of St. George's Hospital and
T. B. Curling. Barnes also helped found the Obstetrical Society of
London and the British Gynaecological Society (two of the societies
that later joined to form the Royal Society of Medicine). He later
personally endowed the first biochemical laboratory at St. George's
Hospital. This was the first laboratory in Britain to measure the
chemistry of blood components and other body fluids to help diag-
nose metabolic problems inside the body.

With a budget of £30 per year, the Board of Management of the
Chelsea Hospital for Women purchased sheets and opened eight
inpatient beds. Occupancy was long then, the first patient being in
for 13 weeks for conservative treatment of prolapse (possibly by

Aveling's sigmoid repositor), while the average occupancy of the hospital was 9.5 women per bed per year. These long stays in hospital may have been made more tolerable by the fact that in the earlier accounts of the hospital supplies, over 10% of the funds for the patients were for wine, beers and spirits. This would greatly upset administrators in our present cost-conscious days in the reformed National Health Service in the UK.

The hospital outgrew the King's Road site and in 1877, only six years after opening, plans were drawn up for better facilities. It was not until 1883 that the hospital moved to the Fulham Road, on the site now occupied by the Chester Beattie Institute. In this decade, the hospital was seeing more than 2000 new patients a year, with over 7000 visits made by women from all over the south of England, from Devon to Kent. Outpatient clinics averaged 50 women at each sitting. Inpatients who could afford it paid a small fee for 'it was believed that by requiring the payment to be made by each patient, feelings of self-respect would not be compromised'. They were charged one guinea a week (payable each Monday) and no other fees were charged except for washing personal linen. The governors of the hospital held an honorary position, provided in return for donating a sum of money to the hospital, and each was entitled to recommend admission of one or more poor women a year. These women were treated in the same liberal way as those who could not pay, but they occupied separate wards; probably two thirds of the women in the hospital were in this group.

In October 1883, the new Chelsea Hospital for Women in the Fulham Road was opened. It was a six-storey building with wards opening off the corridor on each of three floors. There was a day room on the ground floor with operating theatres and staff accommodation above the wards. Outpatient numbers rose and more medical staff were appointed to the hospital. They were allocated only one bed each, being paid no salary but living on the fees of their private practice. At first they attended the respectable poor in the outpatients department and assisted their seniors in their operating theatre. Perhaps the most notable to join at this time was Sir Thomas Spencer Wells. Trained at St. Thomas's Hospital, he had served in the Royal Navy as a general surgeon and was elected a Fellow of the Royal College of Surgeons while working at Bighi Naval Hospital in Malta. He served throughout the Crimean War, in which he gave great service to the wounded. On his return he specialised in the new discipline of gynaecology and devoted the rest of his life to the speciality. By the time he joined the Chelsea Hospital in 1883 he had already performed 1000 oophorectomies. In the same year W. H. Fenton was appointed as the first anaesthetist to the hospital. It might be suggested that fewer skills were then required in anaesthesia, for two years later he was reappointed to the hospital as part of the gynaecological surgical staff where he served with distinction for 30 years.

In 1894 John Bland Sutton joined the consultant staff. As Bonney described it: 'It was fortunate for me that at Chelsea Hospital for Women, where I went as a resident officer in 1898... the banner of Surgery was flaunting there, chiefly owing to the presence on the honorary staff of one – that remarkable man, John Bland Sutton, who brought inspiration to all who worked alongside him, and who rose, solely by his own industry and genius, from very lowly beginnings to worldwide surgical celebrity. This appealed to my young imagination as something heroic.' [2]

Bland Sutton was a man of great energy; he was one of the general surgeons of the hospital and so was allowed to operate on women abdominally. He later served as president of the Royal College of Surgeons. Bland Sutton was a dextrous abdominal surgeon and a forceful character, one of the men who made gynaecology a specialist subject and influenced many young surgeons. He was a great hero of Bonney's and was a major influence leading him into gynaecology. Bonney and Comyns Berkeley joined Chelsea Hospital for Women at about the same time, and Bland Sutton had a great influence on them both. Interestingly, Bland Sutton was also an admirer and friend of Rudyard Kipling and appeared, lightly disguised, in several of the Kipling short stories.

'The honorary staff, in accordance with the custom of the time, was divided into surgeons and physicians, though there was not much difference in the work they did. Bland Sutton and Arthur Giles were the surgeons and William Duncan, Hugh Fenton, Inglis Parsons, Thomas Watts Eden, Ewen Maclean and Comyns Berkeley the physicians. Every branch of our profession becomes intensely interesting when you know enough about it, and when that knowledge is reinforced by the inspiration flowing from a great teacher it becomes enthralling – even to obsession. I determined to become a gynaecological surgeon.' [2]

In 1899 Bonney was employed by the hospital, first as a house surgeon and then as a resident medical officer (RMO) on a salary of £50 per year. He published his first scientific paper in the *Lancet* on August 5, 1898 on 'The After-Treatment and Post-Operative Complications of Coeliotomy for Pelvic Disease in Women'. This was his review of the postoperative course in '200 to 300' women who had laparotomies for gynaecological symptoms. Bonney analysed each, gave excellent clinical observations and tried to out-line the physiological causes of each woman's symptoms.

William Duncan asked Bonney to volunteer to be a surgeon in the army for the Boer War that had recently broken out, but he did not wish to do this for he felt it would loosen his hold on the pro-motion ladder that he was just beginning to climb. Another impor-tant consideration was that Bonney had very swiftly fallen in love with a night sister at the Chelsea, Annie Appleyard, whom he described as having pretty hands and feet. She was from Tasmania, one of four daughters of a doctor, all of whom had come to Britain to become nurses. Bonney proposed and became engaged to Annie.

It was at this time that Bonney decided to take the Mastership examination in surgery (MS) at the University of London, which he passed (Figure 5). The century passed with no great notice from Bonney and Annie, and he then took his final FRCS in October 1900. The most notable thing seems to have been his worry about the examination fees, which were 15 guineas, an equivalent then to three private patient assistant fees. At the same time William Bonney, Victor's father, sat and passed the Edinburgh FRCS. An unrecorded and unknown incident occurred at about this time lead-ing to a distancing of William Bonney from Annie. This led later in life to Annie looking unfavourably on all the younger members of the Bonney family (except of course for Victor).

After an attack of septicaemia following a sore throat, Bonney went to Leicester to convalesce. He reports that he rode with the Quorn Hunt (a most uncharacteristic thing for him at the time). After returning to London, Bonney continued this interest in the aristocratic sports and would often go to the National Sporting Club to watch the evening boxing bouts. He returned to the Chelsea Hospital in April 1902 much refreshed, but realising even then the old adage that gynaecology was for the seniors while obstetrics was for the junior doctors, he sought for and found a place at Queen Charlotte's Hospital.

'I went from Chelsea to Queen Charlotte's Hospital as resident to equip myself in obstetrics, though even then I had determined not to undertake private midwifery, holding that it was not the province of a consulting obstetric surgeon.' [2]

Queen Charlotte's Hospital was situated in the Marylebone Road, and Bonney worked hard there, making a point of becoming friendly with the then labour ward sister, Miss Bacon (whom he privately considered to be a dragon). With his recently found accomplishment of conquering examination hurdles, he took the MRCP, his third higher diploma, and passed that also on the first occasion.

'Obstetrics and gynaecology were...loosely attached to the Royal College of Physicians, membership of which was then a *sine qua non* for all appointments, but I do not think that the College was ever very enthusiastic about the connection, and tended to become less so as gynaecology became "surgicalised".' [2]

In the February of 1901 Bonney stood with his father in a house in Piccadilly watching the funeral of Queen Victoria. This coincided with the passing of an era and the end of British supremacy in the world, although recognition of this did not come to some until after the First or even the Second World War.

'Then came the first of the three big strokes of luck which have befallen my surgical career, for in 1901 Ewen Maclean went to Cardiff and I was elected onto the honorary staff of Chelsea Hospital for Women to fill the vacancy; as a physician mark you, a title I agitated against and presently changed to surgeon.' [2]

By now Bonney had left Queen Charlotte's Hospital and was doing private teaching in order to make a living. He had no other income until elected obstetrical tutor to the Middlesex Hospital, where he wrote on the pathology of puerperal fever. This post would not allow him access to beds to admit a case, but it was a another rung on the specialist gynaecological ladder to full honorary consultancy. Bonney took his first consulting rooms at 10 Devonshire Street to see private patients. At this time Annie resigned from the Shoreditch Hospital for health and family reasons.

The Boer War finished with a British Pyrrhic victory after the loss of many men. Gone were the days when wars were fought on open plains with red-coated soldiers lining up against each other in formation. The guerrilla methods of the Boers taught the British Army that there were ways of fighting other than marching columns of men straight at the enemy. A peace treaty was agreed at Pretoria between Kitchener and the Boers on May 21, 1902. At home, Edward VII's coronation had to be postponed because he had an appendix abscess that required surgery.

Annie moved to London to work, firstly at St. Bartholomew's Hospital and later at St. George's Hospital (at Hyde Park Corner) and whilst there, lived in the Annie Nation Nurses Home in Montpelier Square. By 1902 Bonney was operating in private practice, mostly in patients' homes and occasionally in nursing homes. He had to provide his own portable operating table, his instruments, sterilising equipment, nursing assistants and anaesthetists. Many of these staff were from the Middlesex Hospital for it was there that he got a registrarship of £20 per year and gave lectures in practical midwifery for a further £20 per year. In his first year he earned £80 from private patients while the rent of the consulting rooms was £100 per year. He had much capital outlay and no money to spare, which may have accounted for the long engagement with Annie.

Two papers on puerperal sepsis were written by Bonney and published in 1902, but the trend towards his real life's work started when he became the Walter Emden Research Scholar in gynaecological cancer investigation. His opposite number as Richard Hollins Research Scholar in surgery was Sampson Handley. Bonney was attached to a cancer ward for clinical investigation of women, and his first research there was on the cytology of papilliferous ovarian cysts. Bonney clearly showed a spectrum of change in cells. This was helpful in making a histological distinction between malignant and innocent papilliferous cysts of the ovary. He met up yet again with Comyns Berkeley whom he knew at Chelsea Hospital, and under whom he had been a student at the Middlesex. They started work together on tubal ligation. Berkeley had qualified in 1891, five years before Bonney. Although at the same medical school, this time interval was a great divide and the two men probably did not meet as students. Berkeley, by now an obstetric registrar and tutor at the Middlesex, achieved a consultancy on the honorary staff of this teaching hospital in 1905 when he was 39. The two surgeons became firm friends and had a long partnership of writing and research. They worked together in perfecting the surgical treatment of cervical carcinoma, Wertheim's radical hysterectomy.

Robert Jones, the orthopaedic surgeon in Oswestry, had just started wearing rubber gloves whilst operating, so Bonney decided to investigate this in the control of potential infection. He added further work on the value of surgical face masks in the limitations of the spread of bacteria. He was staying up until two or three o'clock in the morning to complete these research studies after a full day of clinical and teaching duties. It was at about this time that Gordon Gordon-Taylor met Bonney and so started their great relationship, both working for a BSc in anatomy. The examination was then held by the University of London; it had two candidates and seven examiners. Bonney remembered that the two would work through the night sustaining themselves with port. Indeed, later in life he claimed that he was kept awake only by bottles of port, a medication that would send most to sleep. They did further research together in the anatomy of mammals at the Zoological Gardens, and both eventually passed their BSc with first class honours in 1904. Gordon-Taylor recalled these days with Bonney:

'Part of this year was spent in the Dissecting Room, part in a crescentic room under the old Lecture Theatre, now no more. I can still hear his [Bonney's] light footsteps across the quadrangle, the rattling of the tray with coffee-pot and cups – the coffee to be warmed up on a tripod over a Bunsen burner, the kick at the door with the summons, "Open the door", when he would enter with a pipe in mouth and a tin of Inderwick Syrian tobacco under his arm, his constant companion and commemorated in the Hospital "Smoker" programme for 1904.

'Taciturnity was the watchword of the night, for night is for sleep or love or other delicious delights; but there were at least two interludes, firstly when he scampered across the hospital courtyard from our lair to catch the 3am post with a letter to his fiancée, the same dogged lover then as he remained for nigh on fifty years of happily married life.' [4]

Bonney and Gordon-Taylor would work most of the night in the anatomy dissecting rooms with Gordon-Taylor doing the dissections and Bonney recording them by the best visual method of the time – drawing. His skills as an artist now came to the fore and the line drawings he made of anatomical and later surgical specimens became legend. Each he signed with the little conjoined initials of

VB with a curl below them. The illustrations were models of clarity which photography of that time could never have reproduced. One of the first occurred in an article in the *Lancet* in 1906 on ovarian resuspension. This is characterised by the VB signature and the presence of the surgeon's hands (ungloved) in the operation drawing.

Bonney gave up private maternity care in 1904 to concentrate on gynaecology, much of it in the oncological field. However he still continued his public work at Queen Charlotte's and Middlesex Hospitals for many years. Indeed, he was called as an expert obstetrical witness in 1920 for a civil case against a practitioner who was unsuccessfully sued for his management of a breech presentation with extended legs and arms. Bonney's detailed account of extended arms shows the practical skills of one who is dealing with these problems and not just pontificating in theory. Bonney's involvement in obstetrics can be gauged by his contribution to both *Ten Teachers* texts, a popular pair of undergraduate textbooks still being published 60 years after their first publication in the time of the First World War. As might be expected, Bonney was one of the chosen teachers from the London Medical Schools in *Ten Teachers in Gynaecology* for this first edition (1917), until the seventh edition in 1942. However, he also was one of the chosen ten in *Ten Teachers in Obstetrics* from 1919 to 1942, remaining a contributor longer than anyone else.

Bonney refined the design of his first major surgical instrument at this time. He was always seeking to save time in surgical operations without cutting corners. The Reverdin needle was a solid shaft with a needle attached. The rigid needle could have its eye opened at the sharp end by a slider, this adaptation being the important addition devised by Bonney. It was notable for the fact that the surgeon passed the curved needle through the tissue in the correct site for suturing, while the assistant placed the catgut through the eye which was then closed and drawn back through the tissues. The assistant tied the knot and the second assistant cut the ends of the knot to the correct length. This allowed the surgeon to place his sutures carefully into pedicles. The speed of the operation was determined by the skill of the first assistant who had to be almost as well trained a surgeon as the main operator. Some found the curved needle rather hard on tissues. Unless passed and withdrawn along a circular route, it could tear the pedicle, but experts like Bonney could use it even for intestinal reanastomosis where very fine sutures were needed. It was a delicate instrument, and could be easily damaged.

A story is told that Bonney, returning home one day where a carpet layer was working, took out his Bonney–Reverdin needle to show the man and demonstrated how it might be useful to sew the seams of carpets together. 'What,' said the carpet layer, 'use a coarse thing like that on one of my lovely carpets? Never!' Bonney, despite this, was a great proponent of the Bonney–Reverdin needle and taught all his assistants to use it properly. The needle was still in active use at the Chelsea Hospital for Women 40 years later when the author became a surgeon there, but the practice has now atrophied, in part due to the increasing use of needles swaged onto the catgut (eyeless needles) which make suturing much easier.

It was in 1905 that the great Ernst Wertheim came to visit the UK. He had performed over 300 radical hysterectomies for cancer of the cervix. Green Armytage, in the book, the *Historical Review of British Obstetrics and Gynaecology* published by Livingstone in 1954, recalls a story he was told by Cuthbert Lockyer. Apparently Lockyer related this account in 1940 at a British Medical Association meeting in Leicester:

Passing through London, Wertheim and Lockyer were invited to dinner by Herbert Spencer. In the course of this social occasion, it was arranged that Wertheim would perform one of his radical hysterectomies to demonstrate the technique. The patient was to be a 63-year-old woman with an intracervical cancer, a patient of Lockyer's at St. Mary's Hospital in Plaistow. A day or two later, an open carriage drawn by a pair of greys was driven by Lockyer down to the country. Spencer of University College Hospital, Appleton Meredith of the Samaritan Hospital and J.H. Targett of Guy's Hospital accompanied Wertheim there. They saw the patient and went into theatre, where Lockyer assisted Wertheim in the operation. Lockyer wore rubber gloves as was usual by this time in surgery but Wertheim would not use them, saying that he would lose his digital sensitivity if he got into the habit of wearing gloves. He started through a midline incision; Lockyer tried to assist by inserting a retractor but Wertheim did not like this as he felt the wounds should only be retracted by an assistant's hands. Wanting further help, Lockyer spotted a young man who had come in and was washing his hands in a corner of the operating theatre, and called to him to come over. Without any questioning Wertheim took the man's hands and placed them to retract the abdominal wound. This the young man did for about one hour during the remainder of the operation.

The sequel of this was sad. The patient died three days later of fulminating peritonitis, the source of which was traced to the young man's bare hands. It seemed that this assistant was a local GP who had come into the hospital to redress a septic wound and had only entered the theatre suite to wash away the blood and pus from his fingers, for that was the nearest tap available. The coroner was not sympathetic. Wertheim went on to Leicester where Walter Tate, a gynaecologist from St. Thomas', asked him if he would call in to that hospital on the way back to Vienna to demonstrate the technique again. Apparently the response was 'No, no, my friend, I will not. I do not wish to leave a bloody track behind me'.

Later, Lockyer went on to report 115 women who had a radical hysterectomy, of whom only 20 died in the perioperative time. Berkeley learned the operation from Lockyer and brought it to the Middlesex Hospital, where his colleague Bonney was not slow to pick it up and refine it. It was in October 1908 that Berkeley and Bonney published in the *British Medical Journal* the first British record of 18 women who had had this operation. There were only two operative deaths, and both surgeons were optimistic about the operation's future.

# CHAPTER FOUR

# GYNAECOLOGICAL
# CONSULTANCY
## *1905–1914*

*If neither foes nor loving friends can hurt you;*
*If all men count with you, but none too much*
RUDYARD KIPLING, *IF*

T he great event of Victor Bonney's life was his marriage to Annie on May 27, 1905:

### BONNEY – APPLEYARD.
*On the 27th May at St. John's Notting Hill by the Reverend J.E.*
*Darling, William Francis Victor, eldest son of William Bonney MD of*
*100 Elm Park Gardens, Chelsea to Annie Oliver, eldest daughter of the*
*late Dr Appleyard, Tasmania*
(*Times* personal notices, May 30, 1905)

The reception was at Potts House, followed by a supper at the Holborn Restaurant. They went to Hyde for a ten-day honeymoon and returned to a ground-floor flat in Manor House, Ladbroke Grove. Here Bonney thought the neighbours rather noisy, although it was a nice place to live. At this time his father was depressed for he had had a contretemps with Bonney's brother Jack, who had attacked him and was actually sent to jail for it. Bonney's other brother, Ernest, having been the resident medical officer at Charing Cross Hospital, was working at Princess Louise's Dispensary, which later became the Princess Louise Hospital for Children. Professionally, Bonney wrote on ectopic pregnancy with Comyns Berkeley, publishing a long article in the *Archives of the Middlesex Hospital* on the history and aetiology of tubal pregnancy. Two of the cases were very early in gestation (19 and 24 days) and Bonney's drawings illustrate the findings of over 6000 serial sections cut longitudinally of the tubes. Not all the drawings were his; many were by ACA – a Miss Appleyard (not related to Annie) who worked as an illustrator for the department of pathology. The authors found little evidence of preceding inflammatory or tubal congenital defect as a cause of the misplaced pregnancy. Bonney, being the obstetric and gynaecological registrar, also published in the *Archives* that year a report of the hospital work done in 1903. Gynaecological inpatients stayed for an mean of 24.7 days and on average 5.3 per week were admitted during the year. There was no inpatient obstetric department at the Middlesex until November 1908, so this account was of the outpatient obstetrics only. It showed that of 619 women delivered, 320 (52%) were by medical students, a great change from modern practice; 158 of these women (26%) were grand multiparae (having had five or more previous babies) and 95 (15%) were over 36 years old. Twenty-one women were delivered by forceps, possibly using the recently invented axis traction models, and no Caesarean sections were performed that year. There was one maternal death (from sepsis) and 15 stillbirths.

That year Bonney did five private operations; his income for these and the year's consultations went up to £450. This was enough to pay the Maples bill for the furniture of the new home. He and Annie dined with friends frequently and his relationship with Berkeley flourished. Bland Sutton had them to dinner in his sumptuous house where the dining room was modelled on Darius' reception chamber in Babylon in 2000 BC. This was a high point for a junior consultant at this time, for Bland Sutton was one of the most eminent gynaecologists in the country.

Bonney was still devoted to opera and he saw Tamagno's last performance in London and Enrico Caruso in *Rigoletto*. This Neapolitan singer had probably one of the most beautiful voices of any tenor in the world, described as 'mellow, sumptuous and of baritone quality in the lower register'. At this time when Bonney heard him, he sang with 'reckless abandon and radiated happiness'. Caruso himself used to describe the ideal tenor as 90% chest and 10% larynx, saying nothing of the brain.

Bonney's love affair with motor cars continued, but he found early models unreliable. Annie, meanwhile, reintroduced him to Kipling's works and he became a devoted fan of this poet, ending up a few years later as vice-president of the Kipling Society.

The Bonneys took a holiday fishing in mid-Wales in 1905 with Maurice du Pasquier, the father of the girl for whom Bonney had had a penchant years before. This holiday was on the river Afon Rheidol in Pumllumon Fawr, staying at a local inn. They visited Aberystwyth a few miles away. About this time Annie started to develop gross anaemia as a result of very heavy menstrual periods. After due consultation with colleagues at the Middlesex and much soul-searching, a hysterectomy was advised. This was probably a sub-total operation, and was performed by William Duncan, the senior honorary gynaecologist and obstetrician at the Middlesex, who requested Sir John Bland Sutton and Comyns Berkeley to assist. All went well at first, but on the tenth day after the operation, Annie developed abdominal pain, vomiting and signs of peritonitis. At first this was treated conservatively, but as the distension was steadily worsening, Bonney apparently suggested to Bland Sutton that a caecostomy be performed to relieve the tension. This was done in the bed on the ward, presumably with a reasonable local anaesthetic. After this Annie made a good recovery. She convalesced first at the Grandsville Hotel in Ramsgate and then at the Bridge Hotel in Llandrindod Wells. This was the sad end of any hopes for a family that the Bonneys had. After Annie's recovery they moved out of the ground floor into a flat at the top of the same building, thus leaving their noisy neighbours and looking forward to a quieter life.

Bonney's professional career was flourishing. He was appointed a Hunterian Professor at the Royal College of Surgeons, giving the Hunterian lectures with coloured lantern slides on puerperal sepsis. He had been made an assistant obstetrical physician at the Middlesex and performed his first Wertheim's radical hysterectomy in 1908. In the same year came his third big stroke of luck, for William Duncan retired prematurely from his post of obstetric physician at the Middlesex Hospital. Berkeley succeeded him and Bonney succeeded Berkeley, again as a physician, a title they at once had changed to surgeon.

At this time Bonney started his collaboration for the great textbook of gynaecological surgery with Berkeley (Figure 6). Textbooks were hard to publish then unless you had made your name, and you made your name by publishing textbooks, so this catch-22 had to be addressed by Bonney. He first produced the illustrations that would be needed for such a technical textbook on gynaecological surgery. These were the famous line drawings characterised by showing the surgeon's hands in the field, thus giving an air of verisimilitude and providing a familiar scale against which the size of the organs at the operation could be judged. Bonney was very proud of his hands and used to describe them as 'the only physical beauty that nature had vouchsafed him' (Figure 7). He therefore used his own hands as the models for these drawings and they can still be seen very clearly in all the editions of his works. The classic illustrations were completed by Bonney while the script was written and carefully checked by both Berkeley and Bonney. The volume went through six editions in Bonney's lifetime and was rewritten after his death by others. In Bonney's editions the dedication reads:

> Those who have taught me and those I taught.
> Those I have worked for and those who worked for me
> Those who have helped me and those I have helped.

As an assistant in gynaecology and obstetrics at the Middlesex Hospital, Bonney had only a few beds in that hospital. In the Chelsea Hospital he was an outpatient surgeon and thanks to the kindness of Hugh Fenton, a much older gynaecological surgeon, he was always welcome to bring inpatients there, using the latter's allocation of beds. Much of his professional work therefore gravitated to Chelsea, which became his alternate Alma Mater for the rest of his professional life.

Bonney, as a friend of Rudyard Kipling, persuaded the writer to address the Middlesex students at their medical school. Kipling's place in literature has undergone a revival of thought now, but before the First World War he was considered an imperialist defender of the Empire and the Establishment – a militant wordsmith. Medical students, conservative to the backbone, loved his ideas, racist and chauvinistic though they were. Kipling wrote and spoke as Bonney thought, essentially a nationalist above all else.

Bonney's private practice increased and teaching had to be reduced in consequence. He went to Edinburgh to operate with James Hamilton, the great Scottish gynaecologist. In 1910 Bonney took £250 in fees and bought a Daimler 15-horsepower car with a three-valve engine. This was to become his delight for many years. Bryan, the night porter at Manor House Flats where they lived, taught Bonney to drive. Although he was a good teacher, Bonney, in this instance, was not a good pupil. Bryan joined the Bonney's domestic staff and stayed on with the family as chauffeur and handyman for 32 years. This included a spell in the Army during the First World War, where he rose to be a major.

King Edward VII died in May 1910. He had matured into a symbol of stability in a rapidly changing world and many, including Kipling, felt his death was prematurely brought on by his efforts for peace: 'he gave his dear life for the safety of a land more dear.' The gathering storm of the coming First World War was over the country and active preparations were being made. Territorial Army (TA) hospitals were being established around the country and all the surgeons attached to these were being given military rank. This, however, did not apply to the gynaecologists despite their then professional bonding with surgery and their mostly being Fellows of the Royal College of Surgeons. Bonney said that he did not join the TA for he felt that his profession was being slighted. He worked on the great textbook with Berkeley and again described their 2am sittings with port to keep them awake.

The National Insurance Act of Lloyd George was in place and Bonney was worried about the effect on the sixpenny dispensaries such as his father had run. The Midwives Act (1910) had established the Central Midwives Board of which Bonney became an early examiner and later a board member. Although he had given up private obstetrics, he was still a regular worker in obstetrics at Queen Charlotte's Hospital and from there published a textbook of midwifery with Henry Jellett, Master of the Rotunda in Dublin. Queen Charlotte's had a reputation for strong, forceful midwives then. The queen bee of the hive was the sister of the labour ward, epicentre of any maternity hospital. She would not allow a doctor to put a foot inside her empire unless she said so, only allowing honorary staff to come under sufferance and positively forbidding junior hospital doctors. Midwifery was her domain and doctors only entered when called. This system was still prevailing in a loose form when the author first worked at Queen Charlotte's in 1960. Bonney disliked the Sister and the feeling was mutual. Other consultants did not stand up to her and maybe this subservience (which Bonney interpreted as cowardice) influenced him in his later feelings toward Carnac Rivett, for example.

Bonney's friendship with Fenton, senior surgeon at the Chelsea, flourished and they often went fishing together. They were remembered for their catches of rainbow trout at Blagdon. He and Annie went down to Cornwall in their holidays for the golf. Sadly for Bonney, this year would be the last of the great Bonney family Christmas dinners when the whole family gathered at lunchtimes and a great singing party would develop all the afternoon and evening.

The coronation of King George V took place in 1911, the same year that the Bonneys moved to 29 Devonshire Place. They took over the whole house, with consulting rooms on the ground floor and the living quarters above. Their staff comprised a cook, a kitchen maid, a parlour maid, a house maid and the chauffeur, Bryan. At this time Bonney's senior colleague, Sir John Bland Sutton, left the staff of the Chelsea Hospital for Women. Being on the Council of the Royal College of Surgeons, Bland Sutton had hoped that such a public divorce from gynaecology might improve his chances of election to president of the College. It worked. The status which arose from being a president of one of the only two Royal Medical Colleges was very substantial in those days, for there was no differentiation in the minds of the public between the political promotion of candidates who had served their colleges well, and surgical ability.

Meanwhile, Bonney went on holiday again in 1912 with Fenton, fishing in Bladair. That year the Gynaecological Visiting Society (GVS) was founded, the first of the major travelling clubs in the subject. The founder was William Blair Bell, an idealist and an iconoclast from Liverpool. This visiting club was founded with the covert intent of breaking the stranglehold that London had on British medicine in general and on gynaecology in particular. Obviously this was not one of the stated aims and so when Bonney was invited to be amongst the first founder members of GVS he accepted readily. The Society has increased in strength ever since and it has been followed by other visiting societies to which it was considered to be a great honour to be invited. Most have about 30 active members only and so a limited number of gynaecologists were chosen. Their original intent was to visit centres of gynaecological excellence in the United Kingdom and overseas, to watch other surgeons operate and discuss their methods. This was in the days before the more frequent scientific meetings that occur now and were the only postgraduate education that many senior consultants could get. Perhaps their scientific function has lessened, but they remain an important social and managerial activity.

Bonney was made a consultant gynaecologist and obtained admitting rights to beds at the Miller Hospital at Greenwich, and was also appointed a gynaecologist to Putney Hospital, two corners of a large triangle, of which the third was the Middlesex Hospital. The geographical disadvantages were tempered by the relatively light traffic conditions in 1912. Bonney used to take his students to both hospitals for teaching and it was about that time that Bonney described how he operated on a woman with an ectopic pregnancy in her home.

The following year Bonney was admitted to the full staff of the Chelsea Hospital for Women. He described his juniors who now worked for him: Stanley Dodd and Bright Bannister. Dodd, a Westminster man, absorbed his surgical apprenticeship with Bonney and went on to be a deft and neat surgeon who held positive views on radiotherapy and developed its use for cervical cancer. He too was one of the authors of *Ten Teachers* through five editions. Bannister was a large man with a gentle personality. Trained at Charing Cross Hospital, he came to Bonney and learnt the skills of traumatic surgery with much manual dexterity and gentle handling of the tissue so as to get excellent results like his master. He later became a consultant at Queen Charlotte's and Chelsea Hospitals, carrying on in the Bonney tradition.

Bonney had a very happy first overseas visit with the GVS to Paris, where he demonstrated the combined use of the Reverdin needle and hand reel of suture material which, while not new, had been re-introduced by him. Bonney also had a knee tray which he took with him so that when sitting down for vaginal surgery with the patient in the lithotomy position, he could put the tray on his knees, cover it with sterile towels and have instruments put upon it. Many surgeons considered this to be a lazy habit and would insist on the sister who was taking the case handing each instrument in turn to the surgeon and then taking it back from him so that he was unclut-tered. Others, like Bonney, thought it convenient to have a place to put those instruments which were used frequently during the oper-ation for ready action. The knee tray has now been replaced by a hook-on tray at the bottom of the table that takes the same position but is a couple of inches above the surgeon's knees and allows him or her to move freely on the operating stool, in contrast to the rather cramped position that Bonney used to adopt with the tray. It was at this time also that he submitted his first major paper on myomecto-my for publication. This described the beginnings of his enormous interest in the conservative surgery of the uterus, which lasted for the rest of his life.

In March 1913, Bonney wrote an article in the *British Medical Journal* on 'The Necessity of Recognising Midwifery as a Branch of

Surgery'. He bemoaned: 'The textbooks of physiology do not deal with this phenomenon of normal labour; the diseases of childbearing find no mention in the lectures on general pathology; the curriculum is divorced from either medicine or surgery and ... there is a separate examination.' [5]

In this article lay the beginnings of the almost lifelong war that Bonney waged to bring obstetrics under the influence of surgeons; in particular he lamented the absence of 'surgicalness' in midwifery, particularly of the lower classes, and compared this with the care of surgical cases; yet both, Bonney contended, had the potential for disaster, particularly in infections and haemorrhage:

'The transgressions against the techniques of modern surgical asepsis [at delivery] is too great to be washed away with a bowl of antiseptic lotion, however diligently used.' [5]

Bonney blamed the lack of prevention of the problem on the profession's attitudes. The concepts of special lying-in and delivery rooms were 'looked upon as academic ideals not to be pressed for in everyday work'. Some of these he considered to be the result of the obstetrical profession's valuation of itself, both in terms of salary (five guineas per delivery) and of professional insistence of their place in relation to midwives.

'The employment of midwives instead of doctors I believe to be a step in the wrong direction ... The establishment of municipal lying-in institutions where women could be attended by their own medical man under circumstances of proper surgical asepsis – they are shadows cast on the present thought by events coming somewhere in the future.' [5]

Perhaps the former thought will not find sympathy in contemporary society, which is accustomed to the midwife now working as an independent practitioner, dealing with most normal cases supported by an umbrella medical care system for problems; the second idea of lying-in beds in hospitals has now mostly come about as Bonney anticipated.

The same year Bonney described in the *Lancet* an operation to replace an absent vagina with an eight-inch length of ileum on its own blood supply. The operation came from R.W. Baldwin in America and had the claimed advantage of helping patients for 'coitional purposes'. This is not Bonney's only etymologic eccentricity – he describes this rather plump girl as of 'stout and cobby build'. As well as describing the techniques Bonney goes into the ethical aspects of coitus without the possibility of childbearing. He declares a human sympathetic view for the woman's point of view, expressing an opinion radical for the pre-war days.

It was just before the First World War that Bonney took part in two very important linked hospital building developments. The Chelsea Hospital for Women was moved from the Brompton Road to a new site in Dovehouse Street in Chelsea, a quiet cherry tree-lined road between the Fulham Road and the King's Road. Following this, Bonney, who had been a Freemason for some years, was put on the organising committee of the Masonic Hospital, and persuaded them to buy the site just vacated by the Chelsea Hospital on the Brompton Road. The Royal Masonic Hospital later moved to Stamford Brook, where it stood on a modern site cheek-by-jowl with Queen Charlotte's Hospital, but it ran into financial problems and is now closed. That year Bonney acquired his first Lanchester car. He and the chauffeur Bryan gloried in its use for gliding across London and took turns to drive the beauty, Bonney with fewer skills than Bryan.

# CHAPTER FIVE

# THE KAISER'S WAR
## *1914–1918*

*If you can meet with triumph and disaster*
*And treat those two impostors just the same*
RUDYARD KIPLING, *IF*

On August 4, 1914, the First World War began. Bonney was 42. From the beginning of the century German industrial power had grown rapidly, and the nation was looking for a world role to equal that of Britain and France. Rumbles had been occurring on the diplomatic scene, for the Kaiser did not like the British. However, a veneer of civility was maintained. At the Kiel Yachting Week in June 1914 two squadrons of the Royal Navy were present showing the flag and the Kaiser (an honorary British Admiral) was dressed in his Admiral of the Fleet (Royal Navy) uniform when he called on the British Admiral commanding the squadrons. Six weeks later the two fleets were at battle stations ranged against each other. The precipitatory factor for the war was the assassination of Archduke Franz Ferdinand, heir to the Austro-Hungarian imperial and royal crown, at Sarajevo in Bosnia in June 1914. The dominoes tumbled from this event following interlinked treaty obligations, and Britain entered the war in August 1914 to help in the defence of Belgium. The night before the war started, Bonney dined at the Savoy with Annie. They sensed a nostalgic mood amongst those dancing for the last time to the beat of the old drum. The general belief, however, was that the war would be all over by the Christmas of 1914. Some were more solemn and recognised a new fading of the sunset in British influence. 'The lamps are going out all over Europe,' said Sir Edward Grey in the evening of August 3, looking out from the windows of the Foreign Office, 'We shall not see them lit again in our lifetime'. This was the epitaph of an established society that would never recover from the loss of men and materials in the years from 1914 to 1918.

The war was the great watershed in the lives of many people at the time. Before it had been Victorian splendour and its Edwardian epilogue, when Britain ruled the world; these had been Bonney's formative years. His habits were set and naturally affected his attitudes and opinions for the second half of his life in the post-1918 world, where Britain was but one of several ex-colonial powers. The country went into economic decline in parallel with the increasing economic might of the United States and the huge manpower of Russia. The gold sovereign went, being replaced by the paper pound note, a simple but symbolic action of devaluation.

Bonney volunteered for the army but was rejected. While general surgeons were welcomed, no one wanted gynaecologists; this showed a large area of unawareness on the part of the service recruiting officers about how gynaecologists were trained. All were general surgeons before having enough sense to specialise in the new field of pelvic surgery. Bonney was promptly informed by Whitehall that 'as the days of Amazons had passed' the State would not require his services. He was crestfallen and envied his surgical colleagues. He missed the uniform, the extra rations and the extra pay. Further, some who were accepted into the Royal Army Medical Corps stayed in their own homes in London for the first years of the war, doing an enormous amount of private practice in His Majesty's time. Later, the experiences of Bonney and Comyns Berkeley in the war years at Clacton-on-Sea showed what gynaecologists could do.

The Middlesex Hospital Board had decided to put at the disposal of the War Office its previous convalescent hospital at Clacton-on-Sea (Figure 8). Here were allocated beds for 110 men and 15 officers as a complete surgical unit with medical and nursing staff from the main hospital. The medical staffing of this unit presented the board of the hospital with problems. Most of their general surgeons were already mobilised or waiting to go to the front. Since Clacton would carry a large volume of major operative work, they could not send one of their physicians as a surgeon-in-charge. Hence they turned to the gynaecological surgeons, Berkeley and Bonney. Both were officially over-age for the armed services, but were asked to volunteer as honorary surgeons in charge of Clacton. Wishing to do their bit, Bonney and Berkeley agreed with alacrity to undertake between them the sole medical and surgical charge of all the patients sent there. This was a heavy medical and surgical load, and the fact that gynaecologists had earlier been turned down by the recruiting officers is ironic when one realises how Berkeley and Bonney spent their war. They 'Boxed and Coxed' at Clacton from

1914 to 1919, with only an occasional escape to the country, usually
to give a lecture: if the speaker was lucky, he could snatch a day or
two away in more peaceful places like Plymouth or Windsor. Bonney
ended one such visiting lecture with the oft-reiterated plea that no
one should open an abdomen who is not competent to deal with
whatever he finds there: 'Thus the gynaecologist is today an expert
abdominal surgeon, especially expert in the pelvis'.

It must be remembered that Clacton was 80 miles from London
at the other end of a difficult railway line. It was almost the nearest
point on the east coast of the UK to Flanders and so was on the very
fringe of the war itself. In daytime the guns could be heard booming
continuously and all night there were half-heard and half-felt vibra-
tions from the same explosive forces. These brought the workers of
Clacton in direct touch with the war. It was sometimes difficult to
sleep at night for the rattle of the window frames from the gun fire,
and the only cure was to keep the windows ajar, quite an undertak-
ing on a cold Essex night.

The story of the Middlesex Military Hospital at Clacton is told
in the *Annals of the Middlesex Hospital at Clacton-on-Sea during the
Great War*. This was written by both gynaecologists, although from
the style, Bonney seems to have contributed more than Berkeley.
The author is indebted to that publication for an entertaining read,
and for the extracts published here.

The two surgeons would each serve a turn for three days, reliev-
ing each other after half a week. During the whole war they were
also able to keep the obstetric and gynaecological departments of
the Middlesex Hospital in London continuing successfully without
intermission. As well as this, both carried on their share of work at
the Chelsea Hospital for Women, and Berkeley was the only consultant member of staff at the City of London Lying-In Hospital for
much of the war. It would be difficult for us to imagine their lives
then were it not for the fact that Bonney left his very full description. He pointed out that they travelled over 40 000 miles during
the war, from Liverpool Street Station (where they used to arrive
two hours before the train was due in order to get a seat), down to
Clacton, two hours away on a good day. The trip was mostly in dark-
ness because the carriages were blacked out as part of air raid precautions, and on occasions air raids stopped the train.

Things were not much more comfortable when they reached the
Clacton hospital. The two surgeons, both of mature age and previ-

ously having led comfortable lives, shared the same bedroom and a communal sitting room, which in daylight hours was also used as a rest room by the administrative staff. Undoubtedly both these master surgeons suffered much physical discomfort in their four years of work for the country. Bonney wrote that the outlook of a medical officer under 25 years of age would, of course, be very different from that of a married one over 40 years of age. He went on:

'Personal comfort, which as a house surgeon we cannot remember being particularly concerned with, in these latter years loomed large on the horizon. Young men can sleep through all sorts of noise, older men are not so fortunate. Nightly peregrinations of orderlies, the cleaning of the theatre and searching under one's bed for the Reds were no doubt very interesting to you, but at times rather high-pitched and prolonged conversations between the night-nurse and the night-orderlies were sandwiched between cries of "Orderly, orderly" from patients in the wards next door and groans from pains and nightmares are not inducive of a hard-working slumber. Again, one's appreciation of food and taste in selecting is apt to intensify with advancing years especially if one's wife happened to be a past-master at the art of catering. However, such things are advantages – we both lost superfluous flesh.' [6]

Published in 1914 was A Guide to Gynaecology in General Practice by Berkeley and Bonney. It was well received for there was practical advice on the situations faced by the general practitioner. No operations were described, but the bias was towards surgical treatments performed by specialist gynaecologists to whom the general practitioners referred their patients. It ran to a second edition three years later.

Bonney and Berkeley used any spare time to write up the results of their radical operations for carcinoma of the cervix, and published their data for the first 100 cases (1907–1912) in the British Medical Journal in 1916. This was the first proper British series. Berkeley and Bonney felt that Britain had a 'characteristic cautiousness' in taking up new innovations and that that was the reason why some surgeons looked askance at radical surgery. Bonney also had time to paint, which had always been a favourite pastime (Figure 9). Harwich, where some of his old residents were serving on board as Royal Navy Volunteer Reserve doctors, was close and he enjoyed going there. He may have met there his friend Kipling who was also a frequent visitor to the naval yards. The light cruiser and destroyer squadrons were also stationed there. Under Commodore Tyrwhitt, these ships took an important role in the battles of both Dogger Bank and Jutland.

At Clacton Hospital the wounded would arrive in convoys of about 130; trains were full of injured men varying from stretcher cases to the walking wounded. The total number that passed though the hospital during the war was 9242; the classified list of injuries and diseases treated is listed in Table 1.

| Injuries and diseases | No. of cases |
| --- | --- |
| Gunshot wounds | 4622 |
| Shell shock | 110 |
| Gassing | 304 |
| Burns | 26 |
| Trench foot | 415 |
| Accidental wounds | 178 |
| Accidental fractures | 140 |
| Local inflammatory disorders | 268 |
| Acute specific fevers | 282 |
| Trench fever and fever of uncertain origin | 715 |
| Diseases of nutrition and metabolism | 104 |
| Diseases of the nervous system | 80 |
| Diseases of the eye, ear and nose | 138 |
| Diseases of the mouth, throat and larynx | 40 |
| Diseases of the lung and pleura | 346 |
| Diseases of the heart | 127 |
| Diseases of the blood vessels | 34 |
| Diseases of the abdomen | 383 |
| Diseases of the urinary system | 220 |
| Diseases of the genital system | 104 |
| Diseases of the joints | 317 |
| Diseases of the muscles | 189 |
| Diseases of the lymphatic glands | 12 |
| Deformities | 87 |
| Lightning strike | 1 |

Table 1

The conditions treated at the Clacton-on-Sea Hospital (1914–1919) [3]

This is a formidable list of conditions that would tax general physicians and surgeons as well as two men who had been, for many of the preceding years, specialists in obstetrics and gynaecology.

Eight hundred and seventy-four major operations were performed by Berkeley or Bonney. Of these, one-quarter were to remove bullets, shell fragments and other foreign bodies, whilst another quarter were to drain wounds. Arterial ligature was performed in 51 cases and the two wandered as far from the pelvis as the common carotid artery and innominate arteries in the neck, the temporal artery in the head and the subclavian arteries in the upper chest. Indeed, they published an article on the treatment of traumatic aneurysms of the subclavian artery in the neck (*British Medical Journal*, 1916). Over five years, the two men operated on the war wounded with only 40 deaths being recorded, remarkably low figures considering the type of cases that came straight off the battlefield with only field dressings to the hospital at Clacton. Some 31 of these deaths were the direct result of gunshot wounds, and only three were from tetanus. Bonney and Berkeley pioneered the use of proflavine in oily suspension for open wounds as a primary treatment rather than day dressings which stuck to the tissues (*British Medical Journal*, 1919).

'I would remind you that at that time the channel ports were unusable, owing to their close proximity to the Germans, and the wounded had to be sent right across France to St. Nazaire, then by ship to Southampton, and then by train to their final destination. Most of our early patients had not had their dressings changed for many days and their wounds were in a condition of deplorable suppuration.' [1]

X-ray examinations were very important, particularly for the location of metallic foreign bodies (Figure 10). A primitive set of equipment was established in Clacton, worked mostly by the two gynaecologists with the intermittent assistance of the Middlesex Hospital radiologist, Dr. Mann, who travelled down for the day occasionally to help them. Common sense, a measuring tape and a pencil were three diagnostic instruments used along with X-rays to localise the surface markings of the foreign body before surgery was performed to remove it. Bonney found time during these surgical duties to write a long article for the *British Medical Journal* (April 22, 1916) on postoperative intestinal ileus, a subject he had explored previously in 1910 in the *Annals of the Middlesex Hospital*. He made accurate observations of the small intestine after surgery showing how a length could be collapsed and nerveless. Above this would be a distended segment, blown up with much gas but little fluid. Above this again was a portion distended with gas and fluid similar to the faeculent material which the patient vomited. Bonney went on to show that relief by incision of the middle gaseous part was useless but drainage of the top section led to relief and saved the life of many patients. He argued in the medical press with his old colleague, Sampson Handley (who had since become a consultant surgeon at St. Bartholomew's) about the rate of relief of the toxic substances. This must have been at the back of Bonney's mind when Annie, his wife, developed postoperative ileus after her hysterectomy and he suggested a line of treatment to her surgeons (Chapter Four).

Bonney followed carefully in the *Times* the account of the retreat of the armed armies from Mons and the Battles of the Marne and Ypres. A static trench warfare set in on the Western Front. The following year, the public's attention was diverted towards Gallipoli and Turkey where the disastrous landings by the Anzac and British troops were blamed on Churchill. As a way out of the stalemate in Europe, it had been envisaged that a seaborne invasion at Gallipoli could gain the heights that overlooked the Straits of Bosphorus. This would allow artillery to deny the navies of Russia the use of the seaway to access the Mediterranean. It was a bold move, but badly planned. The naval improvisation was good, but the Australian, New Zealand, French and British troops had to land on open beaches under heavy Turkish fire from the shoreline and the cliffs above. There was no port to land supplies. The campaign ended some months later in failure with the withdrawal of the troops and Churchill in disgrace. Possibly, Bonney thought, many of the hard thoughts the Australians had in later years about the 'Poms' dated from this campaign. In the North Sea, the battle of Dogger Bank resulted in the sinking of the German cruiser *Blücher* by the Royal Navy, probably the greatest and most heavily armed fleet in the world at that time. Bonney describes an evening when, dining with Fenton at George Street, the first Zeppelins appeared over London; the whole dinner party was out on the pavement watching them. In that raid, Fore Street in the City was bombed and Bonney saw the searchlights picking out the cigar-shaped enemy airships high over the town.

The war led to a shortage of young doctors, for on qualifying they were immediately signing up to go to the front. Their absence from junior hospital posts and postgraduate training soon became apparent. Senior house officers (SHOs) at the Middlesex became rare and Bonney once had an argument with Ferguson as to whether to take women as house surgeons. Bonney took the opposite point of view, and instead felt that the alternative of taking Indian SHOs was a wiser plan. He was still 'Boxing and Coxing' with Berkeley with three-day stints of residential duty at Clacton, where he oversaw the buying, for £10, of a secondhand de Dion Bouton car for the Military Hospital. This was an invaluable addition to the transport fleet at Clacton and did good service ferrying nurses and patients to the railway station. Later they borrowed a charabanc (Figure 11).

When in London, Bonney used to take great pleasure in visiting the Empire Theatre. He saw Basil Hallam in the first performance of Gilbert the Filbert and the Byng Boys backing George Robey as a lead comic. However, the more serious side of life dominated. There were food shortages in Britain, and the Irish Rising of 1916 distracted attention from the war against the Germans. The Battle of Jutland took place off the west coast of Denmark and Bonney, along with many other British people, took a great interest, deploring the lack of deck armour protection on the heavy cruisers of the Royal Navy, which suffered many casualties. Admiral Beatty was in charge of the battle cruiser squadrons when six battle cruisers were reinforced with four ships from the Fifth Battle Squadron. Beatty was heavily criticised for the way he treated his ships – almost as a wing of cavalry from the Civil War 300 years before, by wheeling them round inside almost impossible circles – but it was he who lured on the German High Seas Fleet until it was under the guns of the British Grand Fleet. There the Germans sustained heavy damage and retreated into the night before they could do even more harm to the Royal Navy. Neither side could claim a victory at the Battle of Jutland, for both sides sustained terrible losses in men and ships, but the German Imperial Fleet never appeared as an effective force for the rest of the war, so in the preventative sense the Royal Navy won.

From his reading of the war Bonney noted the staggered release of news, often being five days behind the events. This allowed for censorship, but the worldly-wise like Bonney also considered the possibility of rewriting history in that interval. He felt that, had the

British public known of the terrible losses on the Western Front, they might have felt a little less jingoistic about continuing the carnage.

Whilst down in Clacton, Bonney also published in the *British Medical Journal* (with C. H. Browning, the bacteriologist at the Middlesex Hospital) the results of his development of the antiseptic solution that his name made famous. He started with Crystal Violet Blue and added Brilliant Green, dissolving 0.5% of each organic dye in 35% rectified spirit, aiming at an immediate sterilisation that also provided an antiseptic state for the duration of the operation. While Bonney originally used this for preoperative cleaning of abdominal skin, its primary use has remained to this day to clean the vagina before vaginal surgery. The solution became known as *Bonney's Blue*. It has been used by two or three generations of gynaecologists to kill bacteria in the vagina before vaginal surgery, for the organic dyes were both antibacterial and antifungal. A further practical gynaecological advantage was the deep purple staining of the whole vaginal surface. This allowed surgeons to know that they had got to the lowest point of dissection at an abdominal hysterectomy; they were below the cervix, and could start freeing the uterus from the surrounding supporting ligaments with impunity. Gynaecologists over the last 60 years have blessed Bonney for providing this moment of relief when, in a bloodstained field, they knew they had at last reached the point where they were certain they were in the safe blue zone of Victor Bonney.

The dyes in Bonney's Blue had high staining capacity. If any got onto the skin or sheets it showed for months and much energy was needed to remove the stain. The story is told of a staff nurse who prepared a patient for operation by Bonney at the Middlesex Hospital. She had painted Bonney's Blue over a large area of the woman's skin, with some resulting spillage on her own hands and forearms. When the patient and her nurse arrived in the operating theatre, the staff nurse showed her stained hands and forearms to Bonney, who told her it would take months to wash off. To the surprise of the surgical staff, the nurse fled weeping from the operating suite. When Bonney asked if this was caused by anything he had said, he was told that the staff nurse was marrying the next day. The operation proceeded, and near the end Bonney slipped out of theatre, leaving his well qualified assistant, George Bancroft Livingston, to close up. When, ten minutes later, Bancroft Livingston left the theatre for the surgeons' room he found the touching scene of

Bonney bathing the staff nurse's hands and arms with cotton wool swabs soaked in ether, an excellent solvent for organic dyes. Victor worked on the nurse to cleanse her of the blue for half an hour to contribute to the happiness of the marriage day. More recently, the English Department of Health raised the issue that Bonney's Blue might be carcinogenic if used in large quantities, but eventually the use of the blue for painting the vagina was spared. Even the mandarins of the Department of Health realised that most women only have a hysterectomy operation once in a lifetime so exposure to Bonney's Blue was limited.

Military conscription started in Britain in 1916. For two years the war had been fought with volunteers to the Army, but the cream of Britain's young men had now been killed or been absorbed into the Western Front from which many would never return. Also in 1916, Field Marshal Kitchener set off for Russia on board HMS *Hampshire*, which was sunk without trace off the Orkneys, probably by a mine. He had been the great hero of the Army from the campaigns of the Sudan and the Boer War to the First World War; he perished in the sinking. Rumours used to exist that HMS *Hampshire* was taking gold to Russia, but this was never confirmed. The drop in morale in the army and the whole country at the loss of Kitchener was enormous.

Bonney's private practice increased, despite the fact that he was only in London for three days a week. He was doing more major operations, increasing his operative experience as well as his bank balance. He was pleased to note that his operative mortality from Wertheim's hysterectomies was better than that of his good colleague Comyns Berkeley, and his operating in private was gradually moving away from patients' homes into Warrington Lodge, a private hospital near Warwick Avenue underground station. However, Bonney as late as 1952 in *Gynaecological Surgery* still included five pages on the preparation of a room for an operation in a private home and the equipment to be transported there.

In 1917 the war moved into the third Battle of Ypres at Passchendaele, where in three months the British army managed to advance five miles, at a cost of 400 000 lives. The United States of America declared war on Germany, partly as a result of the planned leak of the Zimmerman telegram by British Naval Intelligence. This implied a Mexican invasion of the USA, and the final straw was the sinking of the US ship *Lusitania* by a German submarine off Cork. At home, bread was rationed for the first time, and Bonney recalled vividly the Silvertown explosion when a munitions factory blew up in Edmonton, North London. The noise was heard 50 miles away in Cambridge. Sixty-nine people were killed instantly and over a thousand injured. Whilst sabotage was suspected, it was never proven.

The last German offensive took place in March 1918, which corresponded with the first major use of US troops in the war. Whilst the US arrival came late to the battlefront, it gave America a seat at the Armistice meeting and a say in the capitulation conditions. The USA, however, played less part in the planning of the new League of Nations in which much faith had been placed. The US Senate would not ratify America's membership, so their delegation had to leave the Peace Congress, for US senators were worried about the potential use of American soldiers in wars involving domestic politics of other countries, particularly in Central and South America. This was despite President Woodrow Wilson's exertions; he had great faith in the League and tried to foster it. He was awarded the Nobel Peace Prize. In actuality, little resulted from the collective security body of the League for it later failed its first two tests against aggressors – the Japanese occupation of Manchuria in 1931 and the Italian annexing of Abyssinia four years later. The war on the Western Front finished on November 11, 1918, but that year was overshadowed for Bonney by the death of his mother, with whom he had been close and had found time to visit most days when he was in London.

In 1919, the Clacton Hospital closed. During the five previous years it had been ruled by a formidable matron, Miss Morgan, who ran the military unit with the two civilian gynaecologists, three sisters, 66 nurses, 40 nurses from the Voluntary Aid Detachment and five auxiliary nurses (Figure 12). The matron was awarded a Royal Red Cross (first class) and two of the sisters the same honour (second class). Three were mentioned in dispatches, but no recognition from the establishment came to the two honorary gynaecologists who gave up their professional practices in London for half the week, travelled under difficult conditions, operated outside their own field and gave to their country an enormous effort.

In this year Bonney published more papers on myomectomy. In the *British Medical Journal* (March 1918) he drew the profession's attention again to this relatively conservative operation, which removed fibroids from the uterus while maintaining the potential for future childbearing. Up until that point, hysterectomy, which involved removal of the uterus, was the common treatment of fibroids – benign rounded masses of fibrous tissue arising commonly in the fourth and fifth decades of a women's life. Bonney considered the disadvantages of the more conservative operation, acknowledging that myomectomy was not a lesser operation and could produce major surgical problems of bleeding, but pointed out that with the then current techniques these risks could be minimised. These he placed against the advantages of conserving the organs of generation:

'Apart from its physical value, the womb has for most women a sentimental value which, however illogical, cannot be lightly dismissed.'

Bonney advocated that the practice of myomectomy should be considerably extended, possibly recalling his own wife's experiences in 1905 (Chapter Four).

At this time Bonney felt that despite what he had been able to do with his surgical experience, subspecialisation was harmful to the progress of gynaecology. He turned his face against any more specialised branches of gynaecology such as gynaecological oncology, despite his being a major practitioner in that field. His ideas on co-operation with radiotherapists were mostly hostile, and chemotherapy for drug treatment of cancer had not yet arrived on the scene. He believed that all gynaecologists should be able to perform the whole spectrum of surgical diagnosis and operations. His private practice flourished and Bonney sometimes used to make comments about the payment of bills in private. It was then usual for consulting room fees to be paid on the spot, often in sovereigns although he did quote one where a patient beat him down to £1 17s 6d. Bonney spoke to the Norwich Medico-Chirurgical Society in October 1918 on 'The Present Position of Midwifery'. He had obviously not revised his ideas on that subject since 1917 and still considered that:

'Obstetrics has been made into a sort of closed borough, and medical students become imbued with the idea that it was essentially different from other branches of the profession.'

Hence, argued Bonney, they would still think like that after qualification and this would influence their thoughts and acceptance of midwives. Bonney was against midwives working alone and thought childbirth should be medically controlled. He gave a graphic, lurid and negative description of the ordinary bedroom as a lying-in room, with its apparent bacteriological dangers. He thundered:

'Delivery was an operation, and when a woman brought forth a child with out assistance she operated on herself.'

Lloyd George ('a tricky and common little man'), who had led the War Cabinet in coalition from 1916, beat Asquith in the general election of 1918 and formed the new Liberal Government. No doubt Bonney's views about the politicking that accompanied this were influenced by Lloyd George's pioneering of the National Insurance Bill a few years before. This Act of Parliament included a contributory scheme insuring the whole working population against the cost of sickness and some of the disadvantages of unemployment. Compulsory contributions were collected from both employers and employees. The first part of this act was mostly about health and was the brainchild of Lloyd George, having beneficial effects on infant welfare and infant mortality. It needed the co-operation of the doctors, which it eventually got despite opposition from the British Medical Association. It actually gave the average doctor a slightly better and more regular income, but did not necessarily improve the finances of the better paid doctors. The passing of the whole act in Parliament raised much opposition generally and among doctors in particular; the latter felt they were being dealt with like civil servants. Each wage earner was urged to resist deductions in their wages as 'a monstrous oppression by the government'.

The Act passed, thanks to Lloyd George's political ingenuity, but it left a bad taste. These manoeuvres had debased the currency of politics, turning it towards direct action rather than constitutional lines. Perhaps one of the first acts of political spin doctoring came into English political history from Lloyd George's 'Ninepence for Fourpence', a powerful slogan and predecessor of the sound bites used as a crude bribe of the electorate. This was furthered by sensationalisation and personalisation of the issues by the popular newspapers and for the first time the media actually swayed opinion. Bonney disapproved of vox populi intruding on traditional Parliament-led legislation. In this Lloyd George did nothing to placate the doctors, all of whom felt they were losing money, for this was the beginning of the salaried service. This political move is now accepted in retrospect by all as the birth of public health and nationalised medical care in Britain, which was one of the first countries to run a state-organised service efficiently.

# CHAPTER SIX

# THE NINETEEN
# TWENTIES
*1918–1930*

*The heat of his spirit*
*Struck warm through all lands;*
*For he loved such as showed*
*'Emselves men of their hands*

RUDYARD KIPLING, *GREAT HEART*

T he years after the war, when Bonney was in his late forties, were greatly enjoyed both professionally and socially by the Bonneys. However, while Bonney felt that many had profited by the war, either financially or in influence and prestige, he felt that he had not been among them. He resented some surgeons who had been in uniform getting what he felt were undue rewards, while he and Comyns Berkeley had worked hard in Clacton with no recognition. Unemployment was high and female franchise added to Bonney's discontent.

Professionally he was becoming even more famous. Many American and Empire visitors were coming to the Middlesex and Chelsea Hospitals to see him at work. Bonney was behind the move that pioneered Chelsea Hospital as one of the first hospitals to open private beds and rooms in special wards of a public hospital; this was closely followed by St. Thomas's Hospital. Bonney thought this was a great idea, for he could have his private patients receiving good treatment from his residents, anaesthetists and nurses whom he trusted. At the same time, while working in the hospital on private patients, he was available for consultation about problems with the public sector. Sadly, that year Bonney stopped doing research for he felt there was not enough time. He found time, however, to speak at the Cambridge British Medical Association meeting in July 1920 on puerperal sepsis; he spoke with great clarity and authority, emphasising surgical excision of infected lesions.

Bonney's private practice moved to 15 Devonshire Place in the heart of London's medical district, where he and Annie lived in style. He presented a paper at the Royal Society of Medicine on 'Maternal Mortality Rates from Sepsis'. He gave an analysis of the Registrar Generals' data for England, Wales and Scotland (1850–1917) showing the major causes of maternal mortality to be sepsis, toxaemia, haemorrhage and embolism. The first is now greatly reduced, but the other three still act as major aetiologies, although they cause a very much smaller number of deaths. After a full analysis of these factors, Bonney again launched into his main thrust – midwifery as a branch of surgery:

'I want to see midwifery not necessarily more operative but more surgical, which is quite a different thing. I want to see it taught and practised as a branch of surgery.'

He regretted not having made more use of his research on reduction of cross-infection by the wearing of surgical face masks, which he had done in 1902. This, he felt, was used by others later, and he had not published the work at the time. This year (1902) he and Annie went for the first time to Banff where his friend Lady Nicholson had a reach of water for fishing. This was to become a frequent and beloved holiday site.

In February that year, Bonney's father died following influenza and pneumonia. He contracted this in the course of his practice and might have recovered, but struggled on because he had an old patient he was determined to save and so worked on into the nights at what he felt to be his duty. William Bonney was buried in Putney Vale Cemetery. This was a wrench for the whole family, but evening singing entertainments started again in due time at 15 Devonshire Place.

The Bonneys had a new domestic staff and were holding formal dinners on many evenings of the week. These were full Victorian functions with multiple courses and accompanied by matching wines; afterwards the Bonneys and their visitors would retire to a nightclub to dance. Bonney was particularly fond of the Embassy Club, which in those days was under the control of Luigi, a talented and famous nightclub manager. There he spent many happy evenings until the 1931 stockmarket crash. He would also visit the Kit Kat Club in Barnes. He attended dinners given at the Trafalgar Inn in Greenwich, but his home in Devonshire Place was his primary focus of entertainment. The Bonneys were presented at Court

(Figures 13 and 14) and at the other end of the social spectrum, George Bonney, Victor's nephew, remembers children's parties held in Devonshire Place where entertainment was tightly ruled by Annie. Victor played squash at the Prince's Club and tennis at the Wimbledon, Ranelagh and Queen's Clubs. He was obviously a very fit man, kept so by his dancing and sport. He would also often walk from Devonshire Place to the Chelsea Hospital for Women across Hyde Park before his operating list, which started promptly at 8.30am. He added horse racing to his social delights, visiting race-courses as far away as Chepstow. He indulged his primary love of fishing, going to Hereford and spinning on the Wye. Later this was to become his major interest. Fishing was also enjoyed in Norway and Scotland that year.

At this time, the Chelsea Hospital Clinical Society was formed. The idea was to allow consultants to demonstrate operations to each other in the afternoon and then adjourn for a formal dinner at the Garrick Club. Bonney enjoyed these gatherings in both their professional and social aspects, as he liked the company of his fellow surgeons. The Society was funded by keeping back the shillings of the guineas from private patients' fees (1 guinea was equal to 21 shillings, so this meant a pound to the surgeon and a shilling to the Society). There were to be three meetings a year and soon an ade-quate fund was accumulated to allow the consultant staff to enter-tain any distinguished foreign gynaecologists who were in town. In turn the three or four senior registrars to the hospital were added as guests. Bonney's name appears frequently in the wide-ranging min-utes, which were kept confidential. At the first meeting he removed 17 fibroids at a myomectomy, provoking serious and light-hearted comment from his colleagues. He was the first to suggest a visitor's gallery in the hospital operating theatre to allow visitors to watch without having to gown up and join the crowd in the theatre. The gallery with its high sloping glass screen persisted to the end of the hospital's life, even in the last revision of the operating theatres of the Chelsea Hospital for Women, when twin theatres were made on the site of an old large one. He also wanted to enlarge the mortuary, but was talked out of this – 'not enough custom'. Not all entries in the minutes were serious. Watts Eden, a senior colleague, com-plained about the colour scheme at Bonney's operations: 'Sheets – green. Stain – violet-blue. Blood – red to purple'. A Chelsea Hospital for Women golf competition was started; Bonney, a non-play-er of golf, went round in 140, thus saving John Blaikley (with 106) from coming last.

In 1922, the Bonneys set off to tour France by motor car. Unfortunately the car broke down halfway through the trip, but Bonney managed to visit many members of the family. On their return Annie was given a Pekinese dog, Fantoy. This was spoiled by both owners and rapidly achieved the status of that well-known syndrome of older dog lovers whose family have left home – the dog became the surrogate of an only child of elderly parents.

Professionally, Bonney sat on a committee on the extension of the Health Service under the chairmanship of Lord Dawson, and published more papers on myomectomy. The following spring (1923) Bonney broke his leg at what he referred to as 'the ankle and higher up'. He had it set and plastered, but three days later was standing on it operating. His list included a Caesarean section and a multiple myomectomy, which would have involved standing for two or three hours. The fracture took many months to heal and he was in a plaster of Paris cast all this time. He visited Ascot, Cheltenham and Chepstow racecourses regularly and voted in the general election when Ramsay MacDonald came to power with his Socialist government. There is little doubt which way Bonney would have cast his vote.

This was to be Bonney's last year as examiner on the Conjoint Qualifying Examination of the Royal College of Surgeons and the Royal College of Physicians. He had liked doing this and thought it was a good clinical test, but regretted what he thought were the attitudes of the candidates coming through, as well as the increase in female doctors. He thought the men attending had less spirit than the women and their ambition became less and less; the calling of medicine he felt had 'sunk to the level of the civil service'. He had no high opinion of women doctors, thinking that they had a less powerful make-up, not just physically but mentally as well. He never held another examinership in the next 15 years of a highly successful professional and teaching life. One wonders whether this is by chance, by his own wish or by the perspicacity of the examination committees, who may have realised he was a man who held extremely strong views about the young generation of doctors coming through, and who was not prepared to bend with the times of the 1920s. All this time Bonney was a civilian consultant in gynaecology to the army.

That year Bonney joined with others in the *Lancet* in an innovation in postgraduate education. The editor (Sir Squire Sprigge, a surgeon) invited distinguished individuals to contribute a series of

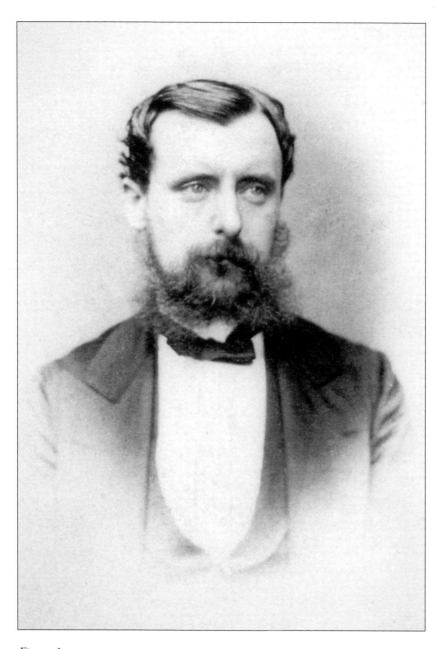

Figure 1
Dr William Bonney, Victor's father, taken at the time of his marriage
to Anna-Maria Poulain

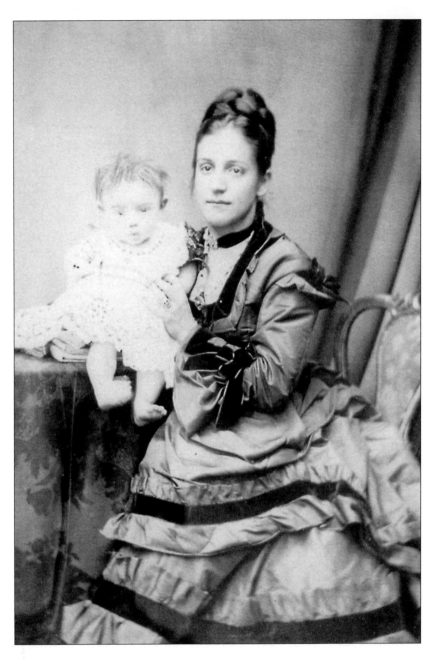

Figure 2
Victor's mother, Anna-Maria, with Victor as a baby

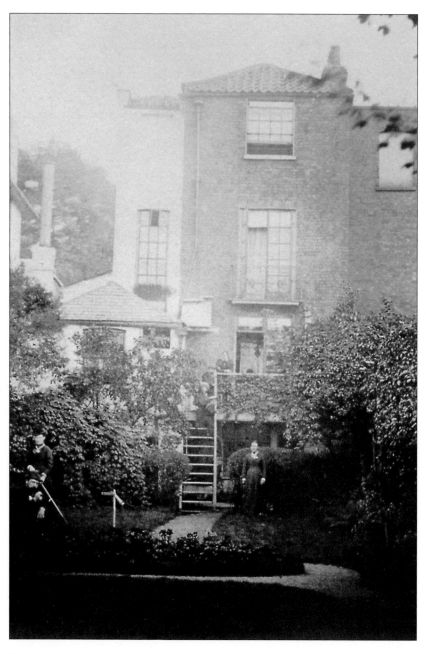

Figure 3

The back garden of the family home, at 320 King's Road, Chelsea. Victor and his two brothers are in sailor suits on the stair, with the nanny at the top. The maid is standing at the bottom of the stair and Dr and Mrs Bonney are seen on the left-hand side

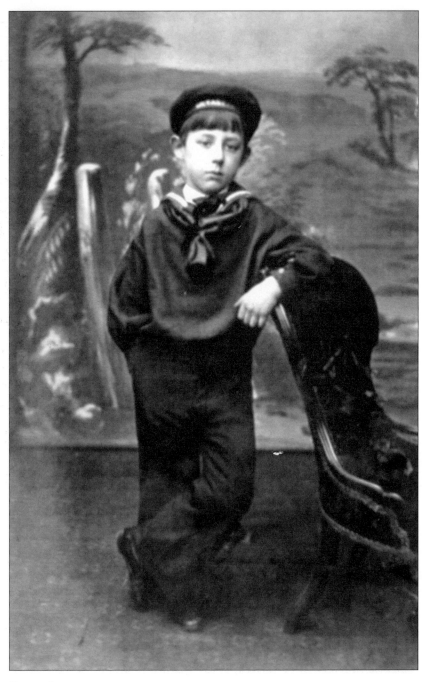

Figure 4
Victor Bonney in 1880

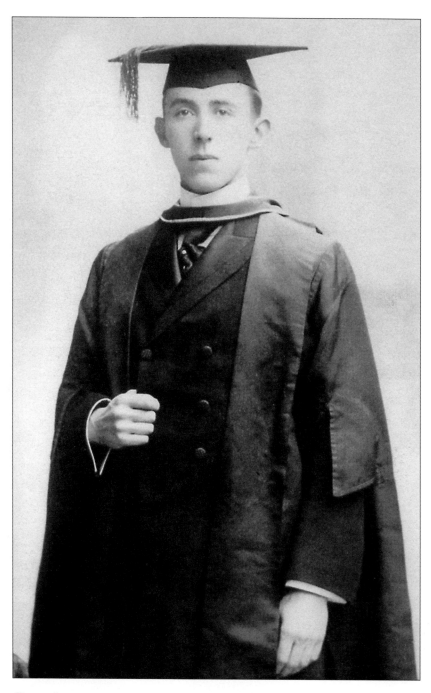

Figure 5
Victor Bonney in 1899 wearing his new Master of Surgery gown

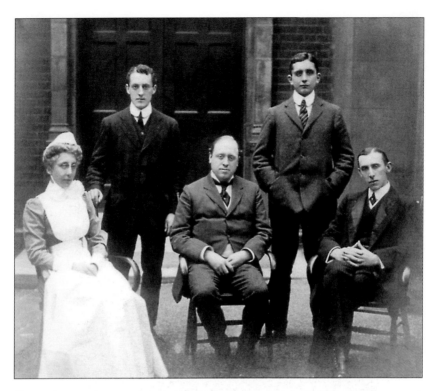

Figure 6
Comyns Berkeley is in the centre with Victor Bonney on the right and their ward sister on the left. The two standing figures were the then house surgeons on the firm at the Middlesex Hospital, 1909

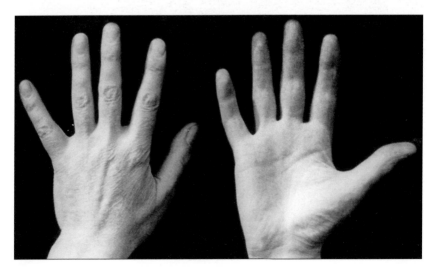

Figure 7
'The only physical beauty that nature had vouchsafed him.' Victor Bonney's hands

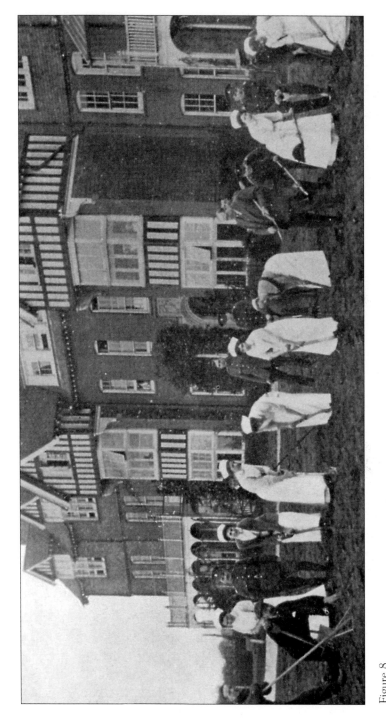

Figure 8
The convalescent home at Clacton-on-Sea with the nursing staff turning the lawn into a potato patch. Comyns Berkeley is towards the right cleaning his spade

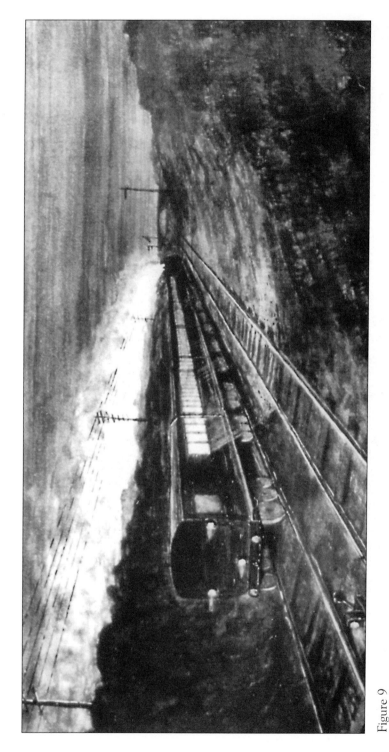

Figure 9
'The Night Express – the Light from the Open Firebox.'
A 1916 watercolour by Bonney

60

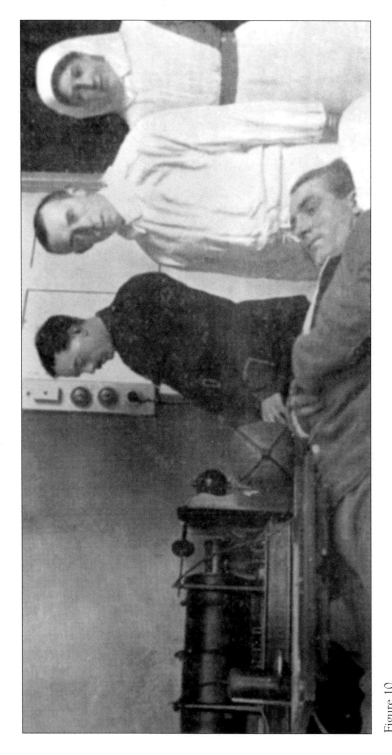

Figure 10
'The X-ray department at Clacton, known as the black hole of Calcutta.' Bonney is seen about to use the primitive equipment to localise a shell fragment

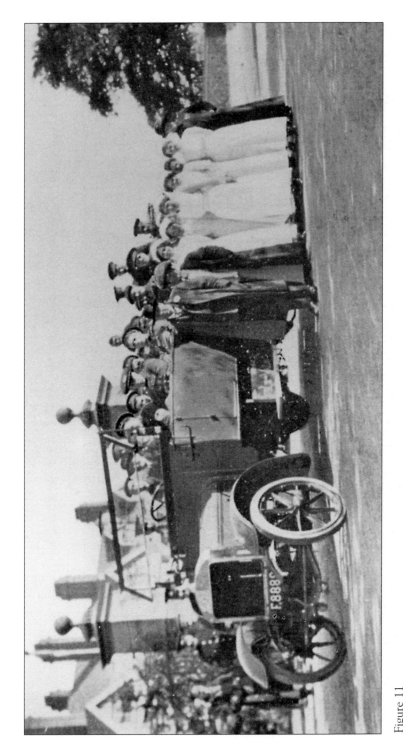

Figure 11
A charabanc leaving Clacton with convalescents on a trip. Comyns Berkeley is to be seen in the foreground

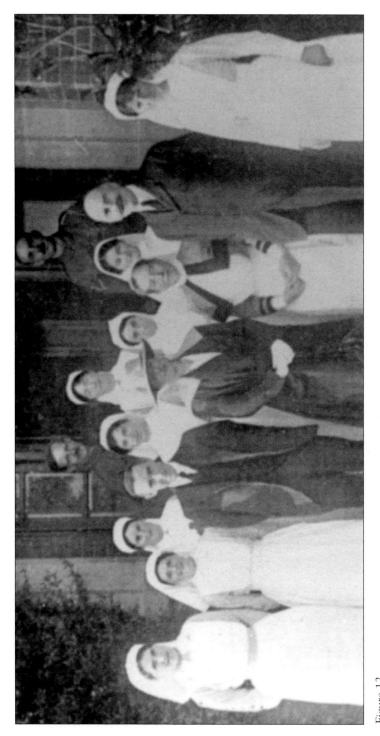

Figure 12
The visit to the convalescent home at Clacton by the Earl and Countess of Athlone (Princess Alice). Bonney is standing on the Princess's right and the Matron is between the two guests

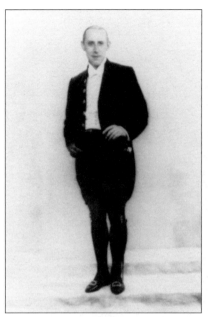

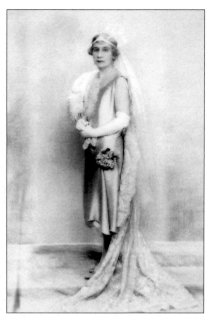

Figure 13
Victor Bonney in Court dress in 1927

Figure 14
Annie Bonney in Court dress in 1927

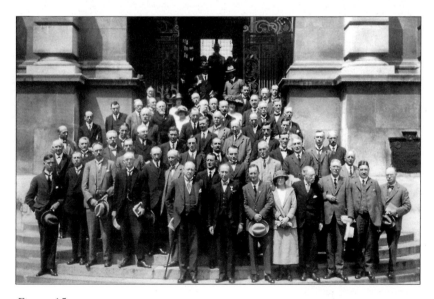

Figure 15
The obstetrical and gynaecological section of the British Medical Association at Portsmouth 1923. In the centre is Bonney, the chairman of the group. Comyns Berkeley is on his right with Fairbairn just behind him. Carnac Rivett is on the extreme left of the photograph

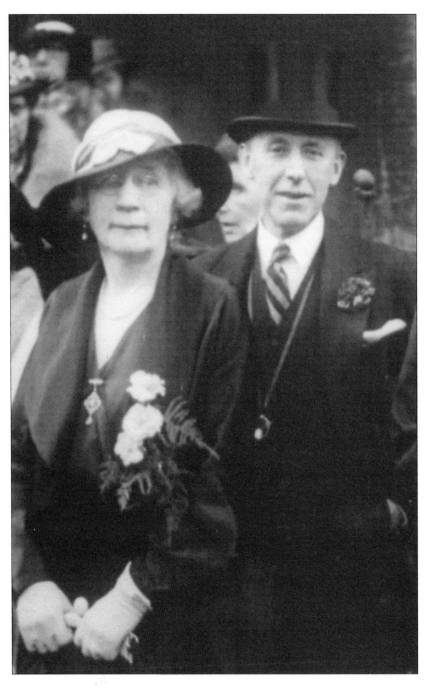

Figure 16
Victor and Annie at a wedding in the 1930s

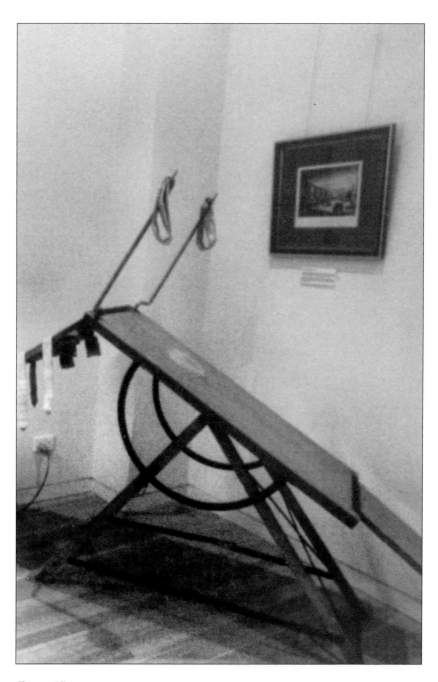

Figure 17
Bonney's portable operating table. Note the steep rake

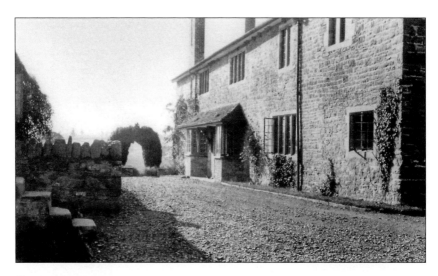

Figure 18
The driveway and front entrance to Seabournes. The main house is on the right and the steps going up to the granary are on the left. The hedge arch leads down to the garden and the River Wye

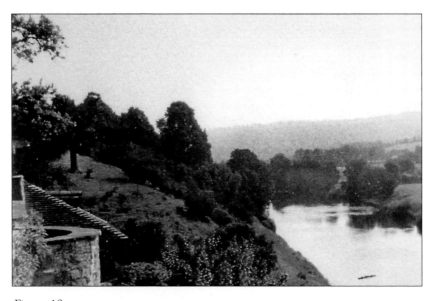

Figure 19
The reach of the river Wye where Bonney greatly enjoyed salmon fishing, seen from the terrace at Seabournes

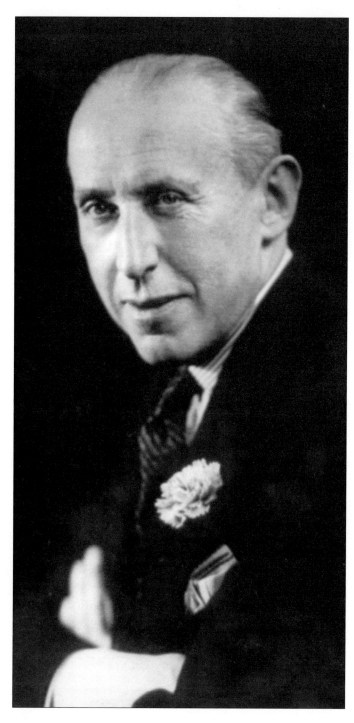

Figure 20
Victor Bonney in 1949

special articles on the treatment of medical and surgical conditions. Bonney was invited to contribute 2000 words on 'The Treatment of Excessive Loss at Periods'. He suppressed his surgical enthusiasm by dealing first with the medical methods then available – ergot and styptics. When these failed (and Bonney hinted they often did) surgery was there to provide a remedy.

The famous myomectomy clamp was also introduced in 1922, an individualistic instrument, which Bonney invented to occlude uterine arteries at each side of the uterus without getting in the line of sight of the operator. It helped to cut off the blood supply of the uterus while allowing the surgeon to perform a myomectomy, a conservative but potentially bloody operation. The myomectomy clamp was uniquely his; others used other devices to reduce the uterine blood supply. Now one rarely sees this clamp in use in the operating theatre, but when one does, enquiry usually shows some directly traceable surgical influence from Bonney's work as a surgeon. The users are third-generation Bonney acolytes, having been trained by his pupils or having worked in one of the 'Bonney hospitals'. The clamp became famous secondarily when it became the emblem of the Victor Bonney Society in later years. This Society was formed by the future specialists, the gynaecological senior registrars of the London and Home Counties regions, for the exchange of views at an annual meeting over a weekend. This included two scientific sessions and a dinner. Members still wear the tie with the Bonney myomectomy clamp as its emblem.

In 1923 Bonney was president of the Obstetrical and Gynaecological Section of the British Medical Association Scientific Meeting (Figure 15). He led in a long discussion on acute salpingitis together with Alec Bourne, Blair Bell and Miles Phillips. Bonney emphasised a surgical approach and justified it, although it was Alec Bourne who was the hero of the meeting with his masterful analysis of the whole problem. In a brief space Bonney published from the Royal Society of Medicine a paper on stress incontinence.

Bonney and Annie travelled to the continent in 1923. They went by train, remembering their motor experience of the previous year. They left a second time that year on a tour of Naples, Pompeii and Sicily, where he objected to the noisiness of certain German tourists who shared his hotels and tour sites. Bonney was generally impressed by Italy and the early effect that Mussolini had had on the services there ('he made the trains run on time'). The following year he visited Glasgow with the Gynaecological Visiting Society (GVS). In his opinion there were only two good gynaecologists in that town at that time – Monro Kerr and Cameron. The former was Bonney's contemporary. After qualifying in Glasgow, Monro Kerr had worked at Chelsea Hospital for Women, returning to Glasgow for the rest of his professional life, eventually holding the Regius Chair in Midwifery. He was a tall man with a mane of hair and a ready sense of humour. Cameron was good at surgery and so was able to be speedy; he repeatedly warned his pupils not to go for speed primarily but let it follow from more skilfully done operations. This was a philosophy that Bonney embraced.

Bonney became disenchanted with the GVS, for although it was supposed to be a scientific group, he felt that the chairman, Blair Bell, allowed no criticism. The meetings were fast becoming mere social gatherings held by Blair Bell. Bonney's attendances at the Society declined after this time and he resigned in the mid-1920s, a most unusual step. His name does not appear among those recorded as attending after 1923, but there is no record in the minutes of his actual resignation. It is interesting that later in November 1937, Bonney was elected an honorary member of the second of the major travelling clubs – the Gynaecological Club. He was the only British gynaecologist ever to be elected an honorary member of that club and was touched by the esteem of his colleagues.

Bonney gave an excellent address to the Windsor and District Medical Society in the December of 1925. He showed he was still skilled in obstetrical matters while discussing puerperal sepsis, stressing the problem of how infection reaches the placental bed after delivery. This, the single biggest cause of death in childbirth in those days, was well analysed and critical management logically laid out. Bonney also spoke about this at the British Congress of Obstetrics and Gynaecology that year when it was held at the Royal Society of Medicine in London. He again stood out for more prompt and extensive surgical drainage. He was the only recorded speaker who considered that the use of rubber gloves at delivery by obstetricians and midwives might be an important innovation. Bonney was instrumental at the end of the Congress in getting an unanimous resolution to go to the Ministry of Health, stating that:

'In the opinion of the British Congress of Obstetrics and Gynaecology, the most urgent requirement in connection with the

problems of [puerperal] sepsis is the provision of adequate accommodation for the reception and treatment of those cases in hospitals, supervised whenever possible by obstetric surgeons.'

Later that year Bonney gave an original paper at the Royal Society
of Medicine with Hugh McEwan, a physician from Belfast, on
'Gynaecology and General Medicine'. Between them they discussed the
general medical presentations of conditions of gynaecological origin. It
was a neat marriage of disciplines, typical of Bonney's active mind.

Also in 1925, the British Medical Association Scientific Meeting
was held at Bath and the Section of Obstetrics and Gynaecology was
presided over by Lady Barrett. Here delegates discussed malignant
disease of the pelvic organs. With Professor Watson of Edinburgh,
Bonney led discussion of surgical treatments. Included was his personal review of 192 cases of radical hysterectomy for cancer of the
cervix. He produced an eloquent panegyric to Wertheim who had
pioneered the operation on the continent and who, Bonney felt, had
not been properly recognised for his service to humanity. He strongly
urged that the operation should be performed by a specialist, stressing that if a surgeon only performed a Wertheim's operation two or
three times a year, he could never become proficient at it. (This
advice the author followed 50 years later when, as a consultant at
Chelsea Hospital for Women, he found himself in that position. He
henceforth transferred all women who needed this operation to a
colleague who performed it about 20 times a year. As well as better
care for the women, this provided more experience for that cancer
surgeon and his team.)

In early 1926, Bonney and Annie went to Egypt via Trieste.
Bonney was fascinated by the Cairo Museum and the Tutankhamun
artefacts that came from Howard Carter's dig. Carter, a self-trained
archaeologist, had been working with the Earl of Caernarfon for
some years; he was convinced the tomb of the young Tutankhamun
was in the Valley of the Kings, but could not locate it. This was the
only Pharaoh's tomb still left undisturbed. After dogged persistence
he found it directly below the tomb of Rameses VI. Since the Earl
was back in Wales, Carter covered up the site, telegraphed him and
with enormous patience awaited his arrival. The *Illustrated London
News* of December 9, 1922 describes how 'the contents include a
royal throne – the first ever discovered – couches, bedsteads, chairs,
chariots, alabaster vases that were so numerous that adequate

arrangements had to be made for their clearance'. The find stirred the imagination of the world, and Carter insisted upon taking the tomb's contents out very patiently in a scientific way. Each piece was photographed, measured and examined *in situ* before it was moved. This was wise, for many of the friable 3500-year-old objects disappeared to dust under the handling of the investigators. In consequence, the definitive examination of the tomb contents took 10 years to complete, during which time, as well as being a scientific worker, Carter had to negotiate with the Egyptian Inspectors of Antiquity, the historical archaeological authorities. All reports were published exclusively in the *Times* or the *Illustrated London News* with other newspapers banned.

In February 1926, when Bonney arrived in Egypt, Carter was just opening the golden coffins of the Pharaoh. Although he does not mention it, since he was in Luxor at this time, it was possible that Bonney was one of the privileged guests who were allowed to go into the inner tomb with Carter and see the work in progress. Large numbers of tourists eagerly awaited the removal of archaeological artefacts from the tomb. Carter continued excavating until the early 1930s and wrote up a very full description of his findings in three volumes, the last one of which was not published until 1932. Bonney met with Fuller, the US Egyptologist from Seattle Museum, who guided him around Karnac Temples and the Valley of the Kings. They then proceeded by train to Aswan and stayed in the old Cataract Hotel, visiting Abu Simbel above the second cataract. They did not go on with the rest of the party to Khartoum, although later in life Bonney regretted this. Tennis was one of his major activities in Egypt and indeed, missing a visit to Khartoum may have been because he enjoyed the tennis at Aswan so much he wanted to stay on playing while the rest of the party explored further.

Bonney and Annie came back by train to Cairo, staying at the Hotel Semiramis. They thought this was a very expensive lodging, but it was nearer the Gezira Club where more tennis could be played. The return to London was via an extended stay in Venice, which impressed Bonney. He studied the history intensively and greatly enjoyed visiting many churches, where he stayed drawing for hours. By the time the Bonneys reached the UK, the General Strike was in progress. The Trades Union Congress (TUC) had promised to back the coal miners if they came out on a general strike. A large force of middle-class volunteers and students was mobilised by the government to keep essential services running, driving buses and lorries to distribute food. The strike was halted after 10 days, for the TUC feared the Home Secretary would legally freeze union funds. Much unemployment followed for many mines and factories closed and stayed so forever.

Bonney's ambition of achieving a position of influence at the Royal College of Surgeons (RCS) was achieved on July 28, 1926 by his election to their Council, gathering 361 votes of the 1100 Fellows who voted. He made a declaration in the terms of the oath pre-scribed by the Charter of 1800 and was greeted at the meeting by his old mentor Sir John Bland Sutton, President of the RCS in his last Council meeting in office. After that meeting, Berkeley Moynihan took the presidency. It was at the same Council meeting that the RCS determined to buy 'for £21, an Imperial typewriter (British made) for use in the Museum Department'. That year, but not at Bonney's instigation, the bylaws of the RCS were changed to allow women Fellows to be eligible to sit on both the Council and the Court of Examiners. The following year Bonney was elected as RCS representative on the Central Midwives Board and to the RCS Discipline Committee and General Purposes Committee.

Bonney's surgical practice was flourishing (see Appendix iii). He operated, not only on private patients but on nearly all the women admitted in his name at Chelsea and Middlesex Hospitals, not pass-ing this work down to his assistants. As well as a full range of gynae-cological and abdominal surgery, Bonney, in common with many of his generation, believed in visceroptosis, the sagging of abdominal organs on their mesenteries leading to pain. He had studied the anatomy of prolapse in detail and devised an operation to make an abdominal shelf; he also added support by suturing the fundus of the uterus to the back of the anterior abdominal wall. He wrote this up in the *British Medical Journal* in 1926 and often included it in what he called his 'round trip' of ventofixation, dilatation and curettage, and vaginal repair. Bonney was still performing general surgery and his ingenuity shows in his simplification of the abdominoperineal approach for carcinoma of the rectum, turning it into a much less bloody vaginoperineal approach. No one but a skilled gynaecologist and surgeon could have thought of this and only the very skilled like Bonney could have performed it.

The next year (1927) Bonney and Annie were invited to New Zealand, to assist in the inauguration of a new society for the advancement of gynaecology and obstetrics. They travelled out via France, Ceylon and Australia, calling at Perth and Adelaide on their way to Sydney. Here, Bonney landed briefly to see Reginald Bonney KC, a descendant of a previous Bonney who had emigrated to Australia in 1834. Reginald was by now a legal adviser to the Australian Government and later was promoted to be High Commissioner in London. The Bonneys then continued their journey on a smaller boat to New Zealand. The trip was a rough one, but Bonney was pleased that neither he nor Annie was seasick, a change from earlier days. He arrived in Auckland in the North Island, which he noted was a mosquito-ridden city, and went on to Hamilton. He operated there on a patient, who unfortunately died on the table. No great blood loss was recorded and Bonney privately considered that in these circumstances the death was attributable to the anaesthetic, but he took the blame. This incident hung like a cloud over the rest of the Antipodean trip. Bonney, like many other surgeons, never liked 'playing an away match on other people's pitches'. He always felt more comfortable with his own operating room with its familiar theatre sister, assistants and anaesthetists, but such was his fame that he was constantly being pressed to demonstrate his operative techniques when he travelled.

Bonney developed a great admiration for the Maori race:

'They were, and still are, a remarkable people; in all respects the finest native race that the white man has ever come up against. Though they have no written script or knowledge of drawing, or understanding of agriculture or manufacture or the art of working metals, yet in the moral qualities of courage, the sense of fair play and straight dealing, they were superior to most whites. Even their cannibalism was a sort of chivalrous acknowledgement, for they believed that by eating the body of their foeman they absorbed into themselves his vigour and courage, which was very complimentary to the gentleman eaten.' [6]

Bonney went fishing in the great lakes of the North Island where he caught 34 trout weighing six to nine pounds each. Both Victor and Annie went further to the South Island where a meeting of the New Zealand Obstetrical Society was held in Christchurch. Bonney was the official delegate of the British Medical Association to the New Zealand branch of the Association. He was presented with an inkstand for the London headquarters as 'a token of the affection and loyalty of the Branch'. This was inscribed with the words, 'Coelum non animum mutant qui trans mare currant' which Kipling translated to, 'They change their skies above them but it is not their hearts that roam.'

Bonney then went on to give a detailed and precise account of 'Genital Displacement', one of the subjects on which he held strong but logical views. The paper should still be read in full by all performing vaginal repair operations (*British Medical Journal*, March 17, 1928:431–3). It is a masterly account of the normal anatomy and variations from this in the pelvis induced by childbirth. He treated the condition as a hernia, applying the same principles of repair as those used in prolapse surgery.

To show that he was an obstetrician also (albeit a surgical one), Bonney also gave an address on puerperal sepsis at the same Congress. He described how sepsis was introduced and then made some profound remarks about Caesarean section:

'Unfortunately nature is inefficient for a certain number of cases and assisted delivery has to take place in spite of the fact that the sepsis rate is a higher one. It should not therefore be resorted to until it is quite clear that the uterus is unequal to the task. The surgeon must take every possible precaution to abrogate the risks that this entry on the operation field entails.'

Bonney goes on to outline those precautions and ends,

'The problem set us is indeed a difficult one, but until it is faced not only by every practising obstetrician but by armchair critics and the State, no striking fall in the yearly death rate from puerperal sepsis can be expected.'

He was an idealist, expecting of obstetricians the same standards as existed in other branches of surgery.

Henry Jellett was an official adviser to the New Zealand Government. He was the ex-Master of the Rotunda Hospital in Dublin and had, a decade before, co-authored a book with Bonney. He had emigrated to New Zealand after the First World War and was highly successful. He had been in dispute with Comyns Berkeley over some professional matter and tried to transfer this debate onto Bonney, who would have none of it. In Dunedin, Bonney addressed the students on the merits of hard work, quoting his favourite poet, Kipling. He went inland to Kingston and Queenstown to fish for salmon. Returning to Wellington, Bonney and Annie set sail for Australia. A strange story exists about a dinner that was arranged in New Zealand for him, but apparently the ship sailed with the Bonneys on board just before the planned date.

Back in Canberra, Bonney, as a Council member of the Royal College of Surgeons of England, took official part in the opening of the new Royal Australian College of Surgeons. He did not think the site was very good, and sure enough the College has since moved to Melbourne. After a visit to Brisbane, the Bonneys returned to Sydney and saw the beginnings of the building of the great bridge, which was finished in 1933. They then travelled on to Hobart in Tasmania and to Longford, Annie's home town, where she still had many relatives and friends. This was her part of the tour; she was coming home after many years. Returning to Melbourne, Bonney addressed the students again on 'The Making of a Surgeon', again quoting Kipling. After this he returned to London for they were worried there might be a boat strike by the dockers. An excellent account of the Bonneys' Antipodean odyssey is written in the *British Medical Journal* (July 21, 1928) and deserves reading to appreciate the sense of Empire that existed between the wars.

Bonney did not enjoy the trip greatly. There was the accidental operative death in the early days of the tour, and Bonney also claimed he was out of pocket by £10 000 for himself and Annie. This was a large sum in the late 1920s. He wrote this off against his duty as a British surgeon and a Councillor of the Royal College of Surgeons to show a mark of respect to the surgeons of Australia and New Zealand and to attend the opening of the Royal Australian College of Surgeons. Nowadays, he would have had expenses paid by the home College as a matter of course. In those days, however, many felt that the honour of representing their College more than compensated for any financial outgoings.

Back in London, Bonney gave an address to the British Medical Association, urging postgraduate training to be organised in Great Britain. He also joined a group of general surgeons in a discussion at the Association meeting in Edinburgh that year on chronic appendicitis. He stressed to the surgeons the need for a proper midline incision for all operations on those with a diagnosis of chronic appendicitis. Bonney pointed out that the 'beautiful little two-inch incision' so commonly used by them did not allow assessment of any major pathology of the pelvis. On the national scene there was a rail strike against the Labour Government, and Bonney considered the financial structure of the country was breaking down, although his private income was higher than ever before.

Bonney attended and took active part in a meeting on the treatment of cancer at the Royal Society of Medicine in London, giving the results of his first 365 Wertheim's operations for cancer of the cervix. Obviously either Bonney or some hardworking assistants had slaved to catch up on the backlog of medical records of the surgeon's work, for 365 is an increase of 172 cases over what was reported at the British Medical Association meeting only two years before. Some 42% of women with all grades of carcinoma of the cervix had cancer cells in the nodes at the side wall of the pelvis. Bonney considered that intravaginal radiotherapy with radium, a new discipline that was increasing in use, could not deal with this. Transabdominal radiotherapy was not yet powerful enough to include the pelvic side walls so all that was then available effectively was surgery. Bonney argued strongly for surgery in combination with radiotherapy. Even in his support for the new discipline, Bonney was determined to make radiotherapy a handmaiden of surgery and not to allow it to become powerful enough to rival his beloved operating:

'Another advantage of radium treatment is that it does not demand of its exponents anything approaching the amount of study and practice needed to become an expert of the radical operation.'

In this same meeting Bonney said that the operative treatment of cervical cancer had 'never been centralised' and so less well trained surgeons operated on patients who 'could have been transferred to the hands of an expert'. This is a very early expression of the cancer policies of the last ten years, in which such referral to tertiary cancer centres is actively encouraged. Yet, this is the man who disagreed with gynaecologists subspecialising in cancer treatment.

The Royal Society meeting provided Bonney with the platform to publicise another of his favourite operations – the myomectomy. By this time Bonney had performed the operation 220 times. He described the numbers of fibroids removed, ranging from one patient with 40 to another with 80. Nor was this a record for Bonney (see Chapter Nine). He described his clamp again, but also described myomectomy during pregnancy, an operation no longer performed for fear of excessive blood loss, which could precipitate the need for a hysterectomy.

In March 1929, the Royal College of Surgeons (RCS) elected Comyns Berkeley to an Honorary Fellowship. Bonney alleged that this was done without his full knowledge, and he wondered whether it might have been in an attempt to help prevent the formation of the British College of Obstetricians and Gynaecologists. Bonney thought that if the Fellowship had been given three or four years before, it might have influenced things, but it was too late now. However, it was granted under the 'twenty-year rule' (whereby the Council of the RCS could consider any doctor for election to the Fellowship after twenty years' membership of the College). It is probable that Bonney's hypothesis that the RCS was seeking to block votes for an independent college was incorrect, for William Blair Bell, the arch-proponent of the about-to-be-launched British College of Obstetricians and Gynaecologists was elected a Fellow of the RCS on the same day under the same rule.

# CHAPTER SEVEN

# THE FORMATION OF THE COLLEGE OF OBSTETRICIANS AND GYNAECOLOGISTS

## *1926–1929*

*Now we are come to our Kingdom,*
*and the Realm is ours by right*
RUDYARD KIPLING, *THE KINGDOM*

G ood ideas often spring spontaneously from several sources. Different people in different places think that something would be a useful thing to do; some keep it to themselves, others discuss it and a coalition may be formed that improves the original idea. Then, occasionally, action is taken on some of these conjoined ideas. So it was with the idea of founding a special college in Great Britain for the management and training of those interested in obstetrics and gynaecology. In the 1920s there were only two medical Royal Colleges in London – the Royal College of Physicians, London (RCP) and the Royal College of Surgeons of England (RCS). There were other medical and surgical colleges in the rest of Britain, but these two were the main ones. Gynaecologists tended to enter their profession through the RCS and obstetricians through the RCP, although the two overlapped and so, many obstetricians and gynaecologists belonged to both.

At this time, it is probable that several people were thinking about, and discussing, the formation of a college in obstetrics and gynaecology, but it was Fletcher Shaw of Manchester who took the lead. He felt the primary objective of a college was to bind the two disciplines and prevent gynaecology from becoming a subdivision of surgery, with obstetrics 'left to those with nothing better to do'. Others held different views, prominent amongst whom was Bonney. He believed that obstetrics and gynaecology would best progress as a faculty of an existing college.

'When I entered gynaecology 55 years ago, nearly all its exponents were obstetric physicians who had learned a certain amount
of surgery, and you may wonder why this was so seeing the part
which general surgery had played in transforming the art. The reason lay in obstetrics which, because it derived from the midwives'
lore in past ages, had always occupied a somewhat anomalous position in the realm of the healing art. The general surgeons of the
nineteenth century suffered from a superiority complex (not at all in
evidence today) and midwifery, because of its feminine derivation
and association, was looked upon with some contempt by all full-
blooded surgeons, though they would have been quite willing to
take over operative gynaecology lock, stock and barrel.' [1]

At that time, gynaecology was primarily surgical in its cures and
so Bonney thought that the subject should be controlled by the
Royal College of Surgeons of England.

'The right remedy as I saw it (and still see it) was for the obstetrician definitely to enrol himself under the banner of Surgery and
to make his spiritual home in Lincoln's Inn Fields, abandoning vain
pretensions to the expert knowledge of a physician, which he never
possessed, and placing himself on the same footing as all other surgeons.' [2]

By this time, as has been mentioned in Chapter Six, Bonney had
progressed to the Council of the RCS, and was putting his ideas forward in the higher courts of surgical thinking. He feared that any
attempt to make a separate college of obstetrics and gynaecology
would widen the gap existing between physicians and surgeons on
one hand and obstetricians and gynaecologists on the other.

'I preached this for years, but my words fell upon stony ground.
To further it [the cause of gynaecology] I became a candidate for the
Council of the Royal College of Surgeons and I think, if time had
been given to me, I should eventually have carried it, though there
was opposition from both sides. But I began too late, for already a
group of North Midland gynaecologists, who disclaimed all allegiance to Surgery, were planning a college of their own, and under
the tremendous drive of William Blair Bell, these men accomplished
it in 1929. It was a very great disappointment to me and I declined
joining the new College.' [2]

Some might put forward less noble ideals than Fletcher Shaw's on the formation of the new College. Those gynaecologists outside the capital resented the hold that Londoners had on the subject and wanted a larger influence in the development of obstetrics and gynaecology. It is of interest to read a letter from Fletcher Shaw (first secretary of the British College of Obstetricians and Gynaecologists) to Eardley Holland in October 1931, saying, 'A weak spot in this College is the large number of London men who have not joined.' He goes on to suggest that the next president should have come from London to rally the ranks of obstetricians there. In parallel with this, outside London the influence of the RCS had been much less and the idea that one had to be a general surgeon before becoming a gynaecologist was not embraced so fully in the country, away from London. Nobody in London thought of going into gynaecology without having first obtained a Fellowship of the RCS and having practised general surgery in the abdomen. This was not so in the provinces, where obstetrics and gynaecology were thought of more as subjects in their own right, so that there was not the instinctive thought of turning to surgery that the London men had.

Fletcher Shaw thought that a body of leading obstetricians and gynaecologists should give weight to the formation of a new college. On the whole, such specialists were individualists and often disagreed with another's ideas just because these were not their own. However, he conceived the idea that the Gynaecological Visiting Society (GVS; see Chapters Four and Six) might be the launching pad for discussion of a college. The Society, founded by Blair Bell of Liverpool, had 30 members, all comparatively young and influential men from various medical schools of Britain, including London. On October 25, 1924, Shaw approached Blair Bell to tell him of his ideas. Blair Bell, a man of wide, acquisitive thought, saw the value of the college and grasped the outlines readily; he also saw the difficulties and wanted to think it over.

In December of that year at the Liverpool MB finals examinations, the two external examiners were Sir Ewan Maclean from Cardiff and Comyns Berkeley. Blair Bell discussed the outline of the plan with them and agreed to bring it to the next meeting of the GVS in Cardiff in February 1925. Bonney was a founder member of that society, but at this time had given up attending meetings regularly. At the Cardiff meeting, outlines of the ideas of the college were agreed, and a small sub-committee was put together to take the matter further. Details of the protracted negotiations for the formation of the college can be found in Fletcher Shaw's book *Twenty-Five Years – the Story of the Royal College of Obstetricians and Gynaecologists (1929–1954)* and are well worth reading by anybody interested in medical politics.

The principles on which the foundation of the college rested were:

(1) to form a portal through which all would pass to be consultants in this branch of medicine;

(2) to prevent the divorce of obstetrics and gynaecology;

(3) to bind together the teachers of obstetrics and gynaecology to allow these to monitor research and teaching; and

(4) to act as a representative body for all obstetricians and gynaecologists.

These ideals may have been modified over the years, but they were the underlying principles. The first one was soon defined so that the entry should be judged both by training in recognised posts in hospitals of the United Kingdom and British Empire and by passing an examination set by the College.

The agreement of the professors of the provincial medical schools was readily obtained. The move to get the London consultants on side extended over some years. Most approved the idea, but some did not agree, prominent among whom was Bonney. The GVS was central to all of this and since Bonney was a staff member of that society he probably received all the papers the various groups were producing.

On October 11, 1926, the RCS started a committee to advise their Council about the advancing threat of the proposed College of Obstetrics and Gynaecology and in parallel moved to consider the question of instituting a diploma in obstetrics run conjointly by the Royal Colleges of Surgeons and Physicians. The small committee consisted of H.J. Waring and V.B. Hogarth, both obstetricians from the London Hospital and members of the Council of RCS, as well as the President and Vice-President of the RCS. Although Bonney was by now on the Council, he was not a member of this committee. One wonders whether his usefulness to the RCS had been overlooked or whether the omission was of his own volition, for he knew all about the preliminary work toward the formation of a College and, although disapproving, he may not have wished to oppose his colleagues in public. In February 1927, the GVS had its last (recorded) discussion in relation to the foundation of the College. This was a meeting in Sheffield, which was not attended by Bonney. It was considered essential to avoid a suggestion that a small elite group of men in a self-elected society should be seen to be founding a national institution, and it was decided that further discussions should be by a wider group of gynaecologists. This meant that from now on no papers about the plans for the College would be circulated to all GVS members and Bonney would lose his database from inside the Society. The GVS had been very important in founding the British College of Obstetricians and Gynaecologists (BCOG). It provided valuable support and a preliminary framework for discussions, but from now on it was a much wider group of consultants who were involved.

In 1927 Bonney wrote a long letter to Fletcher Shaw urging the maintenance of obstetric standards:

'There is no reason why the change of status in obstetrics and gynaecology should not coexist with a College of Obstetricians and Gynaecologists provided that College was itself in favour of such a change, but would it be? However, my private views will not deter me from doing the best I can to help you Fellows who are keen on it. I consider myself your representative on the Council of RCS and as such pledge to do all I can to help you.' [7]

By 1929, however, Bonney's attitudes had changed. It might be that this was catalysed by a secretarial blunder in the organisation of the BCOG. Just before the College was founded, the names of those elected to the first Council were announced to the *Times*. By an oversight, Bonney's name had been included in this list without his knowledge or consent. Adding insult to the apparent injury, he was described as 'Doctor', a title which suggested humble links with general practice. This was the final straw. Bonney was outraged and immediately sent a stiff note to Blair Bell:

'I have, however, to complain that I received your invitation on the morning when the *Times* announcement appeared in which was included my name. I think you will agree with me that there was some fault in procedures and, that I ought to have been given the chance of considering the invitation before any public announcement was made.

'As a criticism of the announcement, which was I suppose approved by the members of Council, I do deplore this use of the word "Doctor" in connection with obstetricians and gynaecologists, at all events in connection with myself, Comyns Berkeley and Rivett who are on the Surgical Staffs of our hospitals.

'I have for years been hoping for the time when Obstetrics and Gynaecology would be accounted as special branch of Surgery and obstetricians and gynaecologists would be considered as surgeons not as physicians, and reading my name among a list which must give to the public the idea of a gathering of respectable apothecaries has fairly made me wince!' [8]

In November 1931, Bonney was again approached to become a Fellow. In his letter of invitation Fletcher Shaw (by now the first secretary of BCOG) said, 'I think you are the only man of any standing who has not joined the College'. In a reply two days later Bonney turned down the invitation, adding, 'I do not express opposition to the College. On the contrary as the large majority of my colleagues welcomed its formation it was quite right to form it and I wish it well and shall always be pleased to further its interest if it comes within my powers to do so.'

To return to the contentious days before this, in 1928 the organisers of the new College had put together a proposal that they hoped would prevent the other Colleges from opposing it. Apparently Royal Charters were not given to an organisation to which there was opposition from another Royal Institution. It was thought that if the College was started as a Limited Liability Company registered with the Board of Trade, it would not have this disadvantage. The word 'Limited' could be dropped later and it was pointed out that many flourishing royal organisations had began under a Board of Trade licence in this way. In consequence, a memorandum and articles of association were drawn up and submitted to the Board of Trade. As was required in such circumstances, advertisements were put in the leading London newspapers announcing this and giving until July 11, 1928 for objections to be lodged. The RCS and RCP kept their countermove until the very last moment. They lodged an objection on July 10, stating that 'the granting by the proposed College of certificates of proficiency in obstetrics and gynaecology would be an infringement of the privileges granted to the two Royal Colleges'. This, in plain language, was the fear of obstetricians trading in on a rich domain whereby the two pre-existing Colleges had received all the fees for the Conjoint Qualifying Examinations in medicine, surgery, obstetrics and gynaecology. The original plans for the new College had not included any wish to take part in or share the fees from examinations at qualifying level, although there were plans for a diploma for general practitioners later on in their professional lives. Having looked at the track record of both the older Colleges in their training plans and qualifying examinations for obstetrics and gynaecology, it is strange that they objected to the new organisation's not even expressed desire of taking this on since education in obstetrics and gynaecology had been grossly neglected by them for many years. It was not until the General Medical Council prodded the RCS and RCP hard at the end of the nineteenth century that they started examining at all in obstetrics and gynaecology, and then very reluctantly.

This rather undignified and late intervention caused an enormous furore, delay and much extra work to all parties. Moynihan (later Lord Moynihan) was by now President of the RCS and Sir Francis Champneys was President of the RCP. Both had been kept informed of the progress of the proposed charter that the new College of Obstetricians and Gynaecologists was seeking. Both had known for a long time that this was being planned but the last-minute intervention caused great disruption and a certain amount of ill feeling between the colleges that took many years to simmer down.

The issue was clouded with many other sub-plots. Some said that the Royal Society of Medicine's Section of Obstetrics and Gynaecology was quite enough for improving the practice of the subject. Bickering went on at various levels between the Colleges for nine months until March 1929, when the Board of Trade held its inquiry.

An unexpected development was a change of government and the Prime Minister's speech putting the reduction of maternal mortality as an important section in his government's manifesto for the next election. This allowed the protagonists of the new College to catch the public eye, and also that of the then Minister of Health, Neville Chamberlain. Brinkmanship continued through meetings of the College Presidents, and on May 16, 1929, things reached an impasse when Moynihan would not accept, on behalf of the surgeons, any of the proposals. It was not until Blair Bell actually got up to leave the room and the debate, so terminating the discussion, that Moynihan asked him to sit down again and, after some further debate, accepted the suggestions. All was not yet resolved, however. Moynihan called a special meeting of the Obstetrical Fellows in the RCS to consider the regulations for a diploma in Gynaecology and Obstetrics. This delayed things further.

Bonney was not party to these latest official discussions, but knew from his position on the RCS Council that a meeting would be held on June 4 that year when the Council of the RCS would discuss the matter. The RCS did not withdraw its opposition, but those steering the negotiations of the new BCOG wisely decided that the Committee planning the regulations for the diploma would not report until after the BCOG was registered. This made things much easier, for there were no official recommendations to consider and so objection could not be made. The President of the Board of Trade accepted the registration on August 26, 1929. Formalities delayed this until September 9, 1929, the date when the British College of Obstetricians and Gynaecologists was actually started.

Bonney had acted with enormous good faith throughout the formative phase and may not have wanted to take a public part against so many of his old friends and colleagues. Indeed, once the College was a *fait accompli*, Bonney refused to act against it and behaved with great generosity towards it. Fletcher Shaw referred to this in his book, saying how Bonney honourably adhered to a policy of 'no public opposition' to the College once it had been founded. Indeed, Bonney even expressed regret later that he had not joined the BCOG governance in the early days so as to have helped mould it.

The first Council meeting of the BCOG was held on September 25, 1929 and amongst the business was the suggestion that they should co-opt Professor Johnson of Belfast, Eardley Holland of London and Victor Bonney of London. The first two of these accepted the invitation, but Bonney declined. The College had other teething problems: for example, many women practitioners were suspicious of a College which they considered to be man-made. In fact, Dame Louise McIlroy had been elected onto the first Council, and of the 218 foundation Fellows, 10 were female, about the same ratio as female to male gynaecologists in 1929. The College soon established itself as the centre of obstetrics and gynaecology, being mainly concerned in its early years with the examination and the co-ordination of teaching in the various parts of the British Isles and the Empire.

Further shots in the all-too-public battle between the colleges came over the Diploma in Gynaecology and Obstetrics, a higher qualification between the level of the qualifying examination and that for the membership (MCOG). It was intended to be a diploma in obstetrics and gynaecology for general practitioners set up by all three Colleges. The RCS held a small committee with four BCOG members on it. Despite this, the BCOG Council considered that if the RCS and RCP did not agree to their joining a conjoint effort then the BCOG should start its own diploma (but not a qualifying conjoint examination). The RCS jumped the gun and started its own diploma, the first examination being held in April 1930. The obstetricians who were examining set a very high standard (roughly that of the MCOG, which was supposed to be for specialists only). Only seven candidates (out of 21) passed the diploma in the 11 examinations from October 1930 to October 1935. As so few candidates passed, the numbers who applied for examination rapidly dropped.

| Examination date | Number of candidates |
|---|---|
| October 1930 | 7 |
| April 1931 | 3 |
| October 1931 | 1 |
| April 1932 | 2 |
| October, 1932 | 1 |
| April 1933 | 3 |
| October 1933 | 0 |
| April 1934 | 1 |
| October 1934 | 1 |
| April 1935 | 1 |
| October 1935 | 1 |

Table 2
Candidates submitting themselves for RCS and
RCP Diploma of Obstetrics and Gynaecology

The examiners on the last three examinations were Fellows of both the RCS and RCP – John Headley, later to become Treasurer of the BCOG, and John Bernard Potts, another founder Fellow of the BCOG. In the last three examinations only three candidates in total applied, each passing the examination. They all came from overseas: Bombay, Cairo and Melbourne. There was a fear that the RCS diploma would be used as a specialist degree overseas instead of the GP examination that had been planned. The examiners themselves recommended that the examination be discontinued, and slowly the Council of RCS agreed. The last examination was held in 1934.

The BCOG started its own diploma in the same year, aiming at the GP who practised midwifery. Originally it was in obstetrics only, but gynaecology was included from the 1970s. Bonney, as a member of the Council of RCS, strongly criticised the decision to stop the RCS diploma. He thought that this would reinforce the ideas of the separation of obstetrics and gynaecology from medicine and surgery, and regretted that surgeons should abandon their interest in this advancing speciality.

It is interesting that 10 years later in February 1939, when the Privy Council was petitioned to request that the BCOG be made a royal institution, no comments were recorded from the Council of the RCS and nothing further was heard. It is also of interest that none of the Royal Medical Colleges of Scotland or Ireland had ever raised any objections to the BCOG formation, nor to its elevation to Royal status.

Bonney went on to become vice-president of the Royal College of Surgeons in 1937–1939, which involved him actively in the affairs of the College. He retired from the Council after his second term as elected member in 1946. In that year, the Council of what is now the Royal College of Obstetricians and Gynaecologists unanimously invited him to become a Honorary Fellow, a high honour. This was because he could not be made a regular Fellow without sitting and passing the membership examination beforehand, a hard thing to expect a retired gynaecologist to do when he was 70. In accepting the honour he acknowledged that the RCOG had not performed as he feared it would. He had fought a long fight to keep gynaecology a subspeciality of surgery. The bond to obstetrics, however, was too strong, and the main subject of obstetrics and gynaecology has since blossomed into its own subspecialities. Strong non-surgical influences have come in as powerful hormone preparations have become more readily available. Since Bonney's time medical gynaecology has flourished.

# CHAPTER EIGHT

# THE NINETEEN THIRTIES
## *1930–1939*

*They took their lives in their lancet hand,*
*And, oh, what a wonderful war they waged*
RUDYARD KIPLING, *OUR FATHERS OF OLD*

Having been a member of the Royal Automobile Club in Pall Mall for years, mostly for the use of the swimming pool, Bonney resigned in 1930 for he felt that membership was becoming too open and he was not attracted by some of the new people who came in. He thought that the Embassy Club too was in decline: Luigi who had run it with consummate grace had died, while Ambrose and his band had moved elsewhere, so Bonney took his patronage to other clubs for dancing. Warrington Lodge, where Bonney had been performing much of his private surgery, declined in quality with the death of the matron Miss Cruikshank, and Bonney transferred his surgical private patients to Manderville Nursing Home, now the Manderville Hotel. This may have been the nursing home depicted in Waugh's *Vile Bodies*. Comyns Berkeley retired and Bonney became the senior obstetrician and gynaecologist at the Middlesex Hospital. Bonney spoke at Berkeley's farewell dinner and this speech is fully recorded in the *Middlesex Hospital Journal* of 1931. As an example of Bonney's humour, this is an account of the old second-hand car they shared while working at the Clacton hospital during the war:

'The clutch would not engage, or, having engaged, would not come out; the brakes had long ceased to be. One day I was sitting in the sitting-room of Miss Morgan, the Matron, when Berkeley had gone out for a run in the car. We saw him pass by the front garden and wave his hand to us, we waved back. After six or seven minutes he passed again and again waved his hand, and we waved ours in return. There was a circular road about three miles long round the town. This took place a good many times, and Miss Morgan said to me: "Mr. Berkeley is enjoying himself!" Presently, round he came again, waving more energetically than ever. We went out, and the car again appeared after six or seven minutes, Berkeley waving frantically and shouting. Apparently the clutch would not disengage, the brakes would not work, and the result was that Berkeley had to go on driving round and round the town because he could not stop. He went round that three-mile circuit 35 times. [Laughter]. If you work it out, it comes to exactly 105 miles!'

For 22 years Bonney had been junior to Berkeley, having only three beds in the hospital. Indeed, if it was not for the generosity of Carnac Rivett, he would never had had enough beds there. Rivett was renowned for his professional kindness. Younger than Bonney and perhaps not so famous, he had got on the staff of Queen Charlotte's Hospital, Chelsea Hospital and the Masonic Hospital just after the Great War. As opposed to Bonney, he was a great proponent of the new BCOG, serving as a member's representative on its first Council in 1929. This philosophical difference of allegiance, however, did not prevent his seeing the real worth of Bonney. Being a most dextrous surgeon himself, he appreciated Bonney's skills in pelvic surgery.

Bonney was re-elected to the RCS Council in 1930 by 514 votes of the 629 Fellows who voted and was made successively Hunterian professor and Bradshaw lecturer there, speaking on puerperal sepsis in the first and on ileus in the second. In each case he opened the eyes of the general surgeons to the fact that an observant, trained scientist in a small branch of surgery could bring new ideas and general principles back to the wider surgical field. Perhaps the most important event of his private life that year was the purchase of Seabournes Farm at Fawley in Hereford, on the river Wye, with three-quarters of a mile of fishing rights on the left bank. Of the original 110 acres, Bonney kept 17 and celebrated his silver wedding anniversary there with Annie that year. In Seabournes much was done on the house and gardens, with a house being built for the chauffeur.

The following year (1931), the country saw a financial collapse in line with much of the rest of the western world. A general election the year before resulted in a Labour victory with 287 seats to the Conservatives' 261 and Liberals' 59. Many, including Bonney, attributed the crisis to Ramsay McDonald. Professionally, Bonney was invited to give a Hunterian oration at the Royal College of Surgeons. This he accepted, giving a great account of himself in radical vaginal surgery for cancer, again striking a blow for the Wertheim's operation and suggesting that radiotherapy was only for the inoperable cases – these would be few in Bonney's hands. He was busy doing the illustrations for the third edition of *Gynaecological Surgery* (published in 1935), but felt that Berkeley did not seem to be very interested in this work now. At the RCS, the Buckston-Browne laboratory at Down House was opened with the idea of emulating Hunter's Farm at Earls Court some 200 years before. Bonney took a great interest in this, serving on the RCS controlling committee. Gordon Gordon-Taylor and Webb Johnson joined Bonney on the RCS Council, making with Sampson Hanley four Middlesex men on the Council, a high local concentration of talent. That year (1931) at the age of 59, Bonney retired from Chelsea Hospital for Women, a hospital for which he had great affection, for he had done well by it and it by him. On November 1932, Bonney took the chair at his last Chelsea Hospital Clinical Society dinner. Dodd proposed his health at length. In reply Bonney gave 'an intimate and interesting account of his long and close association with Chelsea Hospital for Women' having come there as a senior house officer at the turn of the century.

The following year Maria and Camilla de Gräfini Graimberg, Bonney's relatives, visited. They were cousins from Germany who were living in poverty under the Nazis. Their grandfather, Karl von Graimberg, had been an important figure in Heidelberg and had saved the Elector Palatine's castle from demolition in the Napoleonic Wars. His portrait is still held by the family at George Bonney's home.

That year Bonney had to stop playing one of his favourite pursuits, tennis, because of the limitations of a tennis elbow. Sadly, too, the singing parties that he used to hold with his brother Ernest and his family stopped. Professionally, Bonney published his new techniques for use at Caesarean section. He showed that once the uterus had been opened, applying traction to the fetal scalp at a lower segment Caesarean section drew the head out in a more gradual way, benefiting the baby and needing a smaller incision in the uterus. Further, he devised a manual compressor to reduce blood loss at the uterine incision. Taking a flattened-out Hodge pessary, he produced a roughly rectangular firm frame, which could be bent slightly to fit the curve of the lower segment. Pressed on the uterus against counterpressure of the fetal head, an almost bloodless field resulted and the uterus could be opened under clear vision. Bonney then fixed side handles to this and had his compressor made by an instrument firm.

By invitation Bonney gave a Bradshaw lecture at the College of Surgeons. He spoke on intestinal problems after surgery, mostly discussing ileus. This was a difficult subject and Bonney thought it was probably above the heads of most of his audience. The same year he was president of the Obstetrical and Gynaecological Section of the Royal Society of Medicine. He spoke and updated his results of radical surgery for cancer of the cervix, showing a five-year survival rate of 41% and a ten-year survival rate of 19%. The operative death rate had been reduced from 20% to 9% in the last 128 women.

Bonney watched while Berkeley was knighted in 1933. The Royal Masonic Hospital, of which he was on the committee, moved to Ravenscourt Park, to a site adjacent to what was then the West of London Maternity Fever Hospital (later to become Queen Charlotte's Hospital in 1940). Victor had been a Mason for many years in the Middlesex Lodge. He never mentioned it in his diaries, but like so many Masons, the philosophy probably permeated his life just below the surface. Once when addressing the Abernethian Society of St. Bartholomew's Hospital, he exhorted the students with: 'Two lines from an old Masonic song spring to my mind: "Antiquity's pride we have on our side/It maketh men just in their station."'[1] A precise knowledge of what Bonney meant is lacking, but the idea of greater human ideals is there.

In 1935 Bonney was becoming a senior among RCS Council members and was more involved in running College affairs. He served on the Finance Committee (one of the elite posts) and Committees of Anaesthesia and Sterilisation. He had also given evidence to the Department of Health Committee on Sterilisation (May 22, 1933).

The Silver Jubilee of George V brought Reginald Bonney KC to London as Australian High Commissioner. He had a flat in St. James from which Bonney and Annie watched the Jubilee procession. That year the American Gynaecological Society invited Bonney to its summer meeting. The Bonneys sailed for America on the *Aquitania*, the great Cunarder, taking with them Annie's new maid,

Elsie. They docked at New Jersey and made the circuit starting in Montreal, going through Philadelphia and Washington and ending at Hot Springs, Virginia. This was, and is still, a large conference hotel set in rolling forest and countryside where the last sunset of Victorian splendour was still shining. White-gloved servants manned every door of the public rooms and opened them before the guests could touch them. Alcohol could not be bought in the hotel for prohibition existed in the state of Virginia and indeed, this was still going on when the author first visited in 1966. As then, in 1936, people brought their own bottle from a liquor store across the tracks and the hotel provided what the Americans called set-ups. After a very good meeting of the American Association of Obstetricians and Gynaecologists, which Bonney addressed, he returned to New York where he operated. Annie was not told of this until afterwards for she was concerned about what had happened in New Zealand a few years before. All went well. There was a great farewell party for the Bonneys at the Rainbow Room and they returned to London in triumph (Figure 16).

That year Bonney was 63 and he sold the house at 15 Devonshire Place and moved into the Langham Hotel, although they were both probably spending more time at their country home, Seabournes, in Hereford. His staff at Devonshire Place had increased to eight servants including a lady's maid, two daily women, handy-man, secretary, nurse and two chauffeurs. Bonney was still doing some operations in private homes; he had two theatre sisters, several sets of instruments and two portable operating tables (Figure 17). They would leapfrog among the houses of the rich and great setting up one operating site and using the Lanchester or the Rolls Royce, each with a chauffeur, to move the other set of equipment and the second theatre sister to the second house where they prepared for Bonney's arrival an hour or so later. Meanwhile, the first team having operated then tidied up, moving to a third house to set up an operating room. Thus Bonney was able to do a lot of work in private homes as well as in the private nursing home at 3 Manderville Place, with consultations at 149 Harley Street.

In the Bonney family, Victor's brother Jack died; George, the son of his other brother Ernest, had entered Eton as a King's Scholar with remission of all fees because of his good marks at the entrance examination. Sir John Bland Sutton also died in 1936, leaving a big hiatus in Bonney's professional life.

In 1936, Bonney's great hero Kipling died. After considerable abdominal pain he had chosen to go into the Middlesex Hospital for treatment because of his friendship with Bonney and Bland Sutton. He was operated on for a duodenal ulcer. Bonney was greatly saddened at the death of a man he had considered the greatest writer in the world for 40 years. George V died just after Kipling, and the King's death was linked to Kipling's by Bonney with the phrase, 'His trumpeter had gone before.' Edward VIII was next to accede the throne, but he had what Bonney and many other establishment figures considered to be a most unsuitable companion, Mrs Wallis Simpson.

Bonney considered the world was in chaos, the League of Nations was powerless, Spain was on the edge of Civil War, and the Nazis of Germany and the Fascists of Italy were obviously going to push for a conflict. In December of 1936 Edward VIII abdicated, preferring his female companion to the throne of Britain. Bonney never thought much of Mrs Simpson. Indeed, he thought that Edward VIII, whom he often met on the social round dancing in the evening at nightclubs, always seemed to choose unsuitable women. There had been several unseemly episodes in public involving the prince, which were described by Bonney as 'smoking, drinking and snogging' at the Embassy Club. Edward had been reprimanded by his royal advisers to set a better example to his subjects. In the end Edward chose to leave the throne and marry Mrs Simpson. Undoubtedly Edward was very much in love with Mrs Simpson and they lived quietly for another 30 years out of the country, but Edward was never reconciled with the rest of the Royal Family.

The following year (1937) saw the coronation of George VI while Neville Chamberlain became Prime Minister. Bonney thought the latter was a narrow-minded man with little knowledge of foreign affairs. This view was shared by many. Chamberlain became the hero, and the villain, of the immediate pre-war period. Having been a Conservative member of parliament from 1918, he had served in turn as Paymaster General (twice), Minister of Health and Chancellor of the Exchequer (twice also). Chamberlain achieved the best success in the second of those three posts. Later, as Prime Minister, he acceded to Italy over the Abyssinia seizure and closed his eyes to the Spanish Civil War. He abandoned the British naval bases in Ireland that had been preserved since before Independence in 1922. These were badly missed in the Battle of the Atlantic against the German U-boats in 1942–1944. Three times in 1938 he flew to Germany and on September 30, 1938 he allowed Germany to annex the Sudetenland from Czechoslovakia. He returned to Britain with the Munich Agreement, a piece of paper telling of 'Peace in our time'. Revisionalists now consider that Chamberlain was buying time for the British defence system to get the country ready for war. In 1938 Britain had very few fighter planes and an ill-equipped army – all the country had was a strong navy.

Chamberlain was undoubtedly associated with the postponement of the Second World War by a year, so gaining time to rearm, but his government was very slow to put into force enlargements in the armament works, and many think that the concept of Chamberlain actively postponing the inevitable war is false. The time gained was fortuitous and not planned – in fact, it was not used to best advantage. It was at about this time that Chamberlain developed carcinoma of the colon. This gave him much abdominal pain and may have accounted for some of his behaviour at this time. Diagnosis was not made finally until a barium enema was performed in 1940. He told no one of it, not even his wife, and it was not until he resigned from the role of Prime Minister in May, 1940 that his closer friends knew of his illness. He died within six months from the cancer, little mourned and with his efforts for peace disregarded.

In 1937, the Bonneys, when in London, were still living in the Langham Hotel. Elective gynaecological operations were diminishing in number as people were leaving London because of the world crisis and the fear of war. Bonney spoke at the Leeds Medical Society on 'The Fruits of Conservatism'. He always considered this to be his best paper and hoped that this side of his work would be that for which he would be most remembered in the future, rather than the radical surgical aspects for which he was so renowned at the time.

Bonney was 65 that year and he resigned from his beloved Middlesex Hospital. He was anxious to avoid tributes and farewell parties, so he walked quietly from the hospital one day, a month or so before the crucial day. He left a note on his desk to the secretary superintendent saying he would not come back. He never returned to the scene of his triumphs, but still used the Woolavington wing for his private work. Bonney often enjoyed lunch in the senior staff room for he took pleasure in the company of his colleagues. James Young, the professor of obstetrics and gynaecology at the Postgraduate Medical School (PGMS), promptly invited Bonney to be an honorary visiting gynaecologist there, working one day a week. The PGMS was new, having been started by Grey Turner in 1935 in an old London County Council (LCC) workhouse. Situated most unfavourably next to Wormwood Scrubs Prison, it was an architectural disaster built to the old LCC Municipal Hospital design. Professor Young was a most patient man who had developed the new department at PGMS with scarce resources and inadequate accommodation. By bringing Bonney into his team alongside V.B. Green Armytage, he strengthened the department's operating and teaching expertise with little expense. Young and Grey Turner, with the later help of people like Ian Aird, the surgeon, and Sheila Sherlock, the physician, turned the PGMS into an international postgraduate centre. Now, as the Royal Postgraduate Medical School, it has burst its original geographical bonds and is taking on land outside. The combined Queen Charlotte's Hospital for Women (comprising the old Queen Charlotte's Hospital and the Chelsea Hospital for Women), which is in the same National Health Service Trust, will move there within the next few years.

In 1936, Bonney had become senior vice-president of the Royal College of Surgeons, spending much more time every day on College work. He was busy at committees and their preparation, for as senior vice-president he was expected to attend every committee, chairing many of them. Bonney always did his homework before each committee so as to be well briefed on all matters that might arise. His record of attendance in 1936 before election to vice-president was 11 of 11 Councils and five of six committees; this rose to 11 of 11 and 55 of 62, respectively, in 1937. As well as the previously recorded committees where he represented the RCS, Bonney joined the *ad hoc* committee to consider the law of infanticide. He did not get on very well with the then RCS president, Cuthbert Wallace.

Bonney became very worried by German propaganda about the invasion of Austria. He feared the war clouds that were gathering, which would inevitably involve Britain in another continental war. Having been a close observer of the First World War and its great loss of life, he dreaded another conflict.

The following year (1938) the Bonneys, with their maid Williams, left the Langham Hotel and moved into a flat at Berkeley Court in Upper Baker Street. Victor was delighted to get back to a domestic environment. However, also in this year his brother Ernest died of heart disease, having had several heart attacks previously. Ernest had been in the London Clinic under the cardiologist Evan

Bedford, where he was charged eight guineas a week which Victor paid. Eventually he died in the Woolavington wing of the Middlesex, having had another cardiac infarction. His family was greatly supported by Victor in later years. There was a debt to the Inland Revenue which Ernest had accrued; Victor paid it for there was not much left in Ernest's estate. Ernest's death came as a catastrophe for his family. With the remains of what he left and with help from her family, his wife Gertrude was able eventually to maintain an independent existence. Her daughter Veronica soon obtained employment. George, who at Eton had done well in the classroom and even better on the river, had obtained a scholarship to go to King's College Cambridge that autumn. This ambition had to be abandoned. Victor kept a benevolent eye on his nephew, showing the flag by going down to Eton with Annie in their chauffeur-driven Daimler on open days. It was through Bonney's intervention with Sir Charles Wilson (later Lord Moran) that George was able to enter St. Mary's Hospital Medical School and to follow his medical studies. It was, of course, coincidental that at the time the St. Mary's Hospital Boat Club was in one of its phases of expansion.

Bonney's professional work continued in private, although the numbers were down. Nevertheless, he very much enjoyed going to the Postgraduate Medical School and to the Royal Masonic Hospital to operate. From June through to September of 1937, however, Bonney was distracted with anxiety about the war. An end came to Bonney's ambitions at the Royal College of Surgeons. Cuthbert Wallace retired and an election was held which passed over the two vice-presidents (Bonney and Grey Turner) in favour of Hugh Lett. Bonney then finished his office of vice-presidency, although he stayed on Council. By now, although he claimed to have no ambition left to be president, he was probably disenchanted not to be suggested for this office for he felt he deserved this distinction. He says he was not disappointed for he felt he was not naturally fitted for such a job as he had so much on his mind there was little to savour and nothing of the job left. This is a change of heart from when he joined Council in 1926, which may have been connected with the creaming off of obstetrics and gynaecology by the BCOG (now 10 years old), so removing much of Bonney's *raison d'être* for working so hard in the RCS.

'My 20 years of close association with the College of Surgeons was very happy, for this great Institution, hallowed by the labour of very many generations of surgeons, all striving within their lights, for a common end, houses the spirit of British Surgery – the living spirit – visibly surrounded, to the mind that has eyes, by a lovely aura of romance, not the airy romance of fairytale and fable, but that far greater romance which Rudyard Kipling saw immanent in all brave enterprise carried through, win or lose, to the very end. The real romance: "What is Thine of fair design in Thought and Craft and Deed/Each stroke aright of toil and fight, that was, and that shall be."[2]

# CHAPTER NINE

# HITLER'S WAR
## *1939–1945*

*If you can force your heart and nerve and sinew*
*To serve your turn long after they are gone*
RUDYARD KIPLING, *IF*

T he phoney war started on September 3, 1939. Much of the attention of the British was diverted to Finland: the Russians had invaded this country and a very gallant but small army of skiing troops was holding them at bay. At Seabournes, Bonney and Annie took in, as an evacuee from London, a young mother with two children who, Victor considered, did not behave very well, but his standards were rather high; 66-year-olds do not stand small children well. Bonney lived in Seabournes and went up to London every week for one day, consulting and operating on private patients. This was the coldest winter for a long time, the temperature at Seabournes dropping to –12°C. The water system burst and Bonney records the subsequent thaw with icicles on the telephone wires. About this time he was made Inspector of Red Cross Hospitals for Gloucestershire and Somerset, involving his having to travel around by road and railways. The trains were cold with the windows blacked out so Bonney could not read. The roads had all the sign posts removed for fear of a German invasion and so local geography was confusing. About this time he began to find his sleep was interrupted. All his life Bonney, like many other active surgeons, had been a good sleeper, taking opportunities as they arose. However, now he started to have frequent dreams about imaginary and fantastic operations where things went wrong. These were so unlikely in Bonney's real surgical career that they worried him enormously.

The German invasion of a series of countries on the continent followed in 1940 and Churchill was made Prime Minister on the resignation of Neville Chamberlain. This was much in line with Bonney's thoughts for he approved thoroughly of the ex-First Lord of the Admiralty. The air raids started, and the College of Surgeons evacuated its paintings to the National Library of Wales in Aberystwyth. Bonney made a visit to the site and reported their good preservation to the Council of the RCS on July 10, 1941. The Royal College's classical collection of historical books went to Shropshire, but the surgical, pathological and anthropological specimens from the Hunter Museum were taken down to the sub-basement of the College and stored in specially reinforced tunnels. In retrospect this was a pity because many were destroyed in the bombing and only a small number of them were left after the war.

A series of Emergency Medical Services Hospitals was opened in the various sectors. The Middlesex was one of these; probably it would have been called a tertiary referral centre these days. Then followed the Battle of Britain, and German planes could be seen over Seabournes heading for the Midlands – Bonney noted there were no British night fighters there. He took on a locum gynaecological consultancy at Cheltenham for the duration of the war in order to release a younger man. He was described by his then house surgeon, Dr Ralph Whiting, as: 'a dapper little man, beautifully but quietly dressed with a double gold Albert across his waistcoat and carrying a gold-headed cane. He charmed all the women (patients and nurses alike) calling them all "Darling".'

In Cheltenham, Bonney performed his record myomectomy – 235 fibroids from one uterus. He surprised outpatient staff by performing very rapid consultations. He would read the doctor's letter, assess the patient (sometimes examining her standing up to save the time of using a couch), tell her what he intended to do and have her out of the room in a couple of minutes, thus getting through up to 30 patients in an hour. This led to 'a lot of eyebrows being raised by the older nurses' and was beyond the understanding of the Outpatient Sister at that time who was used to more leisurely country hospital activities. His speed at operating was notable also, working on numbers of cases not known before. Bonney had his own operating pyjamas washed and ironed at home and carried in a green cloth satchel. He used to remove his teeth and put them in a glass before operating.

As a part of his peregrinations around the Red Cross Hospitals Bonney met again with Queen Mary. He recorded on this occasion that he had met her previously, but there is no record that Queen Mary was ever a patient. His favoured nursing home, 5 Manderville Place was damaged by bombs, but the London Clinic (his alternative operating site), and 15 Devonshire Place (his consulting rooms), were unaffected. Comyns Berkeley also suffered from several episodes of bomb damage. Bonney kept up his peripatetic West Country Red Cross inspections, while continuing his work at Cheltenham and his one day each week in London. After a day's operating he would spend the night in town, and a bedroom for him was kept at the Royal Masonic Hospital. His house surgeon would then telephone Seabournes at seven o'clock every night during the rest of the week to report progress. The Council of the RCS took him to London monthly and he attended eight of the 11 meetings that year.

Bonney was much concerned with the war, and it occupied his mind. He followed the African campaigns to and fro across the desert, the sinking of the *Bismarck*, and the Russian campaigns, and often worried about the bombing. The fourth edition of *Gynaecological Surgery*, published in 1942, was mostly prepared by Bonney alone for Berkeley was not doing very much now. Bonney was greatly saddened by the death of Hugh Macrea to whom he had given his beloved billiard table when he left 15 Devonshire Place. Civilian bombing of the capital reduced and with the consequent return of people to London, private patients' consultations increased. It was in this year (1942) that a bronze bust of Bonney was crafted by Elsie Pentland. It was exhibited at the Academy and won the Glechen Prize for the best work on show by a female sculptor. There are two copies of the bust in existence now, one in the home of his nephew George Bonney and the other at the Royal College of Obstetricians and Gynaecologists, where it is displayed each year for the annual Victor Bonney Lecture. It looks magnificent when lit on a plinth on the stage, and appears on the cover of this book with RCOG permission.

The Royal College of Surgeons was badly damaged by bombing and Webb Johnson, by then President, reckoned that funds to the value of £2.5 million were needed to restore it. Bonney again took a part in inspecting the RCS pictures that had been evacuated to the National Library of Wales in Aberystwyth and reflected on these art treasures which might have been destroyed had the decision been left to the College. He took the opportunity to do some fishing in Wales. This was the last year he went to Banff to fish, for Lady Nicholson was getting old, and this was another break with the past. Bryan left the service of the Bonney family in 1942, having been with them for 40 years. Bonney had a little house built for him just outside the gates of Seabournes, and Headley Joyce joined as the new chauffeur. The war had now spread to the Pacific and this concerned Bonney greatly, but he followed with an active interest in all the campaigns that were going on.

In May 1943, Bonney delivered a Hunterian oration at the RCS on 'The Forces behind the Specialisation in Surgery'. He laid down that obstetrics was a branch of surgery:

'Of all the departments of surgery, obstetrics is perhaps the most surgical, for pregnancy is a state induced by the rapid growth of a neoplasm; natural labour is to be regarded as the operation which the woman performs herself, and when the obstetrician has to intervene he does so with his hands or his instruments. It is surprising therefore that for many centuries, so operative an art should have been allowed to wander disconsolately between the confines of medicine and surgery.'

Again, the ability of the surgeon to deal with every condition that may be confronted during surgery was stressed, and Bonney frowned upon the need to call in another surgeon. In this lecture all these hobby horses were reinforced by such considerations as Neolithic flint axe heads, Plato's philosophy and Bonney's favourite poet, Kipling.

By now the British College of Obstetricians and Gynaecologists was actively applying for a royal charter. Bonney criticised the College's structure and management privately, but said nothing in public that might hurt its chances of royal recognition. The following year Bonney started writing his great book on myomectomy, doing this whilst on duty at night in the hospitals. Food was short and he was amongst the grateful recipients of food parcels from the American Gynaecological Society, the generosity of which was recognised by many gynaecologists in this country during the war. He was also glad of parcels from his relatives in Australia. Berkeley developed intestinal obstruction and was operated on by Webb Johnson, an extremely fine surgeon. However, Berkeley requested that Bonney should be present also. There was a ring stricture at the splenic flexure of Berkeley's large bowel. This could have been removed, but Bonney records that Berkeley had insisted before the operation that it would not be so because he wanted to be out of hospital very quickly to look after his wife who was mentally unstable. Hence a bypass was performed, and Berkeley did very well.

In the winter of 1944, the Council of the RCS records a letter from the Royal College of Obstetricians of Gynaecologists (RCOG) suggesting that the three Royal Medical Colleges (RCP, RCS and RCOG) should be housed on one site after the war. This would allow common lecture theatres, libraries and domestic areas, but a separate floor or even a wing for each of the three medical colleges. The Surgeons agreed provided the site was in Lincoln's Inn Fields where there was plenty of space. The Physicians did not agree, saying they would never leave Trafalgar Square (they moved to Regent's Park later). These were insuperable difficulties. Doctors in this country could have had a strong unified Academy of Medicine in 1945, but they disagreed and soon it was too late. The War Claims Repatriations money was spent elsewhere and many new colleges and faculties flourished, so that by 1994 there were 18. Bonney would have despaired.

# CHAPTER TEN

# AFTER THE WAR AND RETIREMENT

*1945–1953*

*Send here the bold, the seekers of the way –*
*The passionless, the unshakeable of soul,*
*Who serve the inmost mysteries of man's clay,*
*And ask no more than leave to make them whole*
RUDYARD KIPLING, *DOCTORS*

T he war in Europe finished in May 1945, and in Japan
in August of the same year; the latter event was precipitated
by the dropping of atomic bombs on Hiroshima and Nagasaki.
Bonney was unhappy for humanitarian reasons, but realised prag-
matically that it probably saved the lives of millions of Allied and
Japanese people, for a prolonged invasion of Japan would have been
very bloody. Already he regretted the loss of life of both soldiers and
civilians during the whole war and the war damage in London. With
the end of the European war, a general election was held and
Churchill, the Conservative leader, was deposed from office, being
replaced by the Labour Chairman, Clement Attlee, as Prime
Minister. Bonney considered this did the country no good at all
overseas and he approved only of one member of the 'gang of Attlee'
– Ernest Bevin, who became a bluff, honest John Bull of a Foreign
Secretary.

In 1946, Bonney buried the hatchet sufficiently to accept an
honorary Fellowship of the (now Royal) College of Obstetricians
and Gynaecologists. He still thought it to be 'run by old women of
both sexes' but felt that the new College (17 years old) was super-
vising the training of young gynaecologists very well so that they
became competent. In 1946 he left the Council of the RCS for the
last time. Comyns Berkeley died that year. His wife had preceded
him and he had packed up home and was being looked after by his
chauffeur's wife. He became more parsimonious in his last days and
died without any family. Bonney always hoped that Berkeley would

have left his quite considerable fortune to the Middlesex Hospital, but he did not, because it was about to be taken over by the government in the forthcoming National Health Service. Instead Berkeley left his money to Caius College in Cambridge. With Berkeley's death, Bonney lost a lifelong companion and friend, someone who had been close to him all his professional life.

The following year (1947), Bonney stopped working at Cheltenham Hospital and the Royal Masonic Hospital. At the latter institution, consultation and operating fees were based on the Masonic applicant's word about his earnings. Bonney sometimes had his doubts that it was the true income that had been declared, and he doubled the level of fees. The Bonneys took a flat in Devonshire Place for the summer in a house that had once been occupied by Dickens. The winter was severe and Seabournes was cut off by floods. Annie required surgery for deformity of the foot, probably a hallux valgus. This was performed by Watson Jones, an eminent orthopaedic surgeon from the London Hospital who had an enormous private practice. He operated, with much improvement of Annie's condition. The Bonneys moved again, leaving Devonshire Place, and took a flat at 155 Weymouth Street. Consulting rooms were rented at the London Clinic. After operating, Bonney used to stay at the flat or in the private wing of the Middlesex.

Tiredness often came earlier in the day for Bonney, who was now 75 and had driven himself hard all his life. He was still a surgeon to be reckoned with, but his work was costing him much more effort. He was tiring easily and often left the closure of an abdominal incision to his assistant. One of his last senior assistants, George Bancroft Livingston, recalls that Bonney would not wear his spectacles to operate, having the idea that he could still see perfectly well. This too slowed things up; Bancroft Livingston used to have to hold the wound open during the operations, for Bonney took a dislike in his later days to self-retaining retractors. Another of his later pupils, Leonard Easton, reinforces the stories of Bonney's poor eyesight and remembers using his hands as retractors to keep bowel out of the surgical field. He also recalls an occasion when Bonney, always fastidious about aseptic technique, called for the scrub sister to give him something to clean out the vagina before starting the operation. He was given a douche bag of water and when he learnt that this was not Bonney's Blue demanded some antiseptic be put in. Apparently for the next few minutes the theatre staff were treated to a bacteriological lecture.

After assisting Bonney at his operations for six months, one of his senior registrars had the temerity to ask if he could perform the next hysterectomy on the list. Bonney looked up from the table and said, 'What, and miss the chance of watching *me* do the operation?' Occasionally, if pedicles were persistently bleeding Bonney would have no hesitation in leaving long-handled artery forceps on with the handles coming out through the skin wound for removal 48 hours later, long after Bonney himself was tucked down in Hereford. No one came to any harm from this but it taxed the nerve of his junior staff. Bonney still walked from his London flat to work and back in his smart suit with an orchid in his lapel, the stem resting in a little tube of water lying behind the lapel.

The National Health Service (NHS) was introduced at this time. Bonney considered the debates were far too much centred on the payment of consultants, and this continued talk of money became distasteful to him. With this emphasis on payment came the idea of a standardised salary to all consultants of all disciplines in the hospitals. This was anathema to many senior doctors. The majority of hospital doctors and general practitioners voted against the Service in a referendum run by the British Medical Association and threatened not to work in it. Aneurin Bevan, the then Minister of Health, was a shrewd practitioner of politics and manager of men. He won over the hospital consultants by allowing them to continue private practice while holding part-time appointments in the NHS hospitals. This was referred to as 'stuffing the mouths of the profession with gold', but was agreed to by the Presidents of the Royal Colleges of Surgeons and of Physicians as being an acceptable way for consultants to behave. In addition, some consultants were awarded distinction awards which, at the highest level, amounted to a doubling of the consultant's salary. At present a third of consultants receive them, and these awards are now much sought after. General practitioners also did well from Bevan, for they negotiated a capitation fee for each patient on their list. It was also agreed that for all new services or treatments coming in after the start of the NHS in 1948, a fee for service would be negotiated. So the profession agreed to join the new Service, and the country moved into the most important social experiment seen this century.

Bonney commented, perhaps a little sourly, on the King's Honours list that year. Gordon Gordon-Taylor and Tudor Edwards both received knighthoods. Bonney cast his mind back to the hard work he had done all his life in gynaecology, his national service to medicine in the First World War at Clacton, his army civilian consultancy for many years and the Second World War years of travelling around the country. It may be that at some point in the past, Bonney had offended someone in the establishment. There was a tale around that he had been consulted by the formidable Queen Mary and, as was his habit, had in the course of his treatment of her addressed the Queen as 'Darling'. This he could well have done and even if he conversed with the King he could have addressed him similarly, for Bonney used 'Darling' in daily talk for everyone. Had this really happened, the Queen would have frozen and stayed icy for years afterwards, but there is no existing evidence of any professional encounter between them.

Carnac Rivett died in 1947; Bonney regretted the loss of this surgeon. He was reportedly critical in the past, saying that Rivett operated by the clock and sacrificed technical safeguards to impress the ignorant. Rivett certainly was a spectacular and rapid surgeon, but actually sacrificed nothing to safety. His technique had been honed down and perfected so he never had to do anything a second time and by this he saved extra minutes. This negative opinion that Bonney was reported to hold of Rivett was uncharacteristic, for he really thought well of the man who had been kind to him earlier in his professional life and of the work he did, and it is probable that he seldom did say unpleasant things about anyone. His nephew George has said that 'gossip and intrigue were entirely foreign to his nature'.

It is interesting that Bonney had in 1947 drawn attention to the great increase in lung cancer amongst men. This was three years before Austin Bradford Hill and Richard Doll produced their classic work on the relationship of lung cancer to cigarette smoking. Bonney, once a heavy cigarette smoker, does not comment on the possible link, although ideas about it were not far away, and it was frequently talked about as an aetiological factor. In his younger days Bonney had also been a great cigar smoker. Many unsubstantiated tales are told of the number of cigars he would smoke in a day, even rising to the improbable number of 50. A cigar every 20 minutes of a 17-hour day would hardly have left much time for operating or consulting. John Blakeley, who was his junior colleague at Chelsea Hospital, is recorded as saying at Bonney's farewell from that hospital that he smoked 12 a day (the first one in the bath in the morning). That is possible but still heavy, for he is also alleged in his heyday to have lit up an ounce of full strength pipe tobacco a day also. Certainly Bonney knew a lot about the keeping and smoking of cigars, but in his last days he stopped cigar smoking and was devoted to his pipe, smoking his very strong mixture only in the garden or his study (Annie's rule).

The partition of India and the declaration of independence of Sri Lanka took place in 1947. Bonney thought this was far too soon for these countries to be given full sovereign status. This feeling was shared by many others, but the Attlee government had made it a point of policy to rid India of the imperialistic yoke. They sent Earl Mountbatten there as Viceroy to do it; Mountbatten was a very efficient naval officer and he accomplished this speedily. In years afterwards many Indians and Pakistanis regretted the speed with which Britain withdrew from dominions that it had helped develop. Religious strife continued for years after partition and is still rumbling on in Kashmir.

Bonney continued his life in the countryside, visiting London one day a week. The Bonneys had made Seabournes much more comfortable and habitable than when they bought it as a simple farmhouse (Figure 18). It had been extended to provide accommodation for the servants and for guests. Opposite the house was a barn, which was known to them as the granary; this had been redecorated and given a new sprung floor. It housed many books and Bonney's own pictures as well as a grand piano. Bonney worked here on many of his drawings and when he invited John Howkins, his last senior registrar, there later in life to consider the illustrations for an eighth edition of the book, it was in the granary that he and Howkins worked. Electricity was provided by a generator that fed batteries housed below the granary. Water was pumped to the house from the River Wye. Later this was found to be heavily contaminated, but nobody seems to have come to any harm.

In the daytime Bonney was never bored; he used to read a lot and loved talking to guests. His conversation was well tuned, and those who joined with him in those days greatly enjoyed his art. He did not play the piano, but he often played selections from his enormous selection of 78 rpm records, which he used to enjoy sitting and listening to, particularly the operatic ones. The *Times* was delivered each day and this he read avidly. The Bonneys had two Pekinese dogs, one of whom had a central disc prolapse causing hind leg paralysis; Bonney had a trolley constructed so the dog could move around propelled by the front legs.

Whilst not overtly religious, the Bonneys used to attend church regularly at the village chapel, St. John's. Annie took a part in the flower rota and church cleaning. There were on good terms with most of their neighbours, but never shot or hunted nor allowed hunting on their land.

Bonney's trips to London were nearly always by train. He could leave Seabournes and pick up the local train at Fawley Station (which no longer exists). This went via Ross to Gloucester where he changed for the London train and within a couple of hours could be at Paddington. Coming back, slip coaches dropped at Gloucester and he was able to make a speedy journey back.

The Bonneys' life in Seabournes was very formal. In the evening, an elaborate ritual of cocktails was prepared; Bonney prided himself on his particular skills in judging the quantity of the ingredients. Then the dressing gong was struck to prepare for dinner, which was always formal with dinner jackets and long dresses. After an interval of about half an hour, the second gong was struck, calling people into dinner. The table was laid with an Omar Ramsden silver service and cut glass. Bonney ate and drank very sparingly by this time, but the quality of the food was excellent, as were the wines. Usually champagne was drunk through the meal, for it was Bonney's favourite wine. After the meal, the port was passed while the ladies were evicted to the drawing room. Bonney never approved of the telling of loose stories. The conversation that went on in the dining room was an extension of his professional and other interests, mostly factual and a little philosophical. After this came the coffee ritual. Bonney was addicted to a Cona apparatus which involved boiling water and passing it under pressure into a glass container filled with ground coffee beans, thus infusing the beans at a high temperature. These were fierce machines but Bonney seemed to have tamed his and it was used with great effect. After dinner they would retire to the granary where Mah Jong was an important part of the evening ritual, taken particularly seriously by Annie. Dancing would take place, with music from a radiogram which had an automatic change, enabling twelve records to be played consecutively. Bonney was still a smooth and neat dancer, moving like a sleek cat through the steps that Annie, his lifetime dancing partner, always followed with perfection.

The gardens at Seabournes were particularly fine, with Annie taking an active interest in their maintenance. She had two gardeners and created a fine flower garden with a hidden kitchen garden behind it. There were many unusual trees in the garden, and the flowerbeds were appropriately changed to suit the season. Fruit was grown there: mulberries, raspberries, loganberries, gooseberries and peaches came to the table. All the vegetables for the house came from there, including excellent asparagus. Far too much was produced for the needs of two people and the few servants, and so the village benefited from the generosity of Annie, who would take produce to the various church fairs and to the people in the village.

The River Wye flowed on the edge of their grounds, providing a fine fishing beat. Bonney was a keen fly fisher in his later years. Salmon were plentiful and the largest fish caught in Bonney's beat was recorded at 26 pounds (Bonney himself had landed a 48-pound salmon in 1925 when fishing at Eden). On March 4, 1951 the last salmon that Bonney landed was recorded in his fishing diary, weighing 16 pounds. He used a Wood Gudgeon spinner, and the salmon was caught in the stretch just below the cottages, to be occupied later by George Bonney (Figure 19). After this, the records of fish caught and reported in the fishing diary has a gap for the rest of 1952, but from then on most of the fish were caught by Joyce the chauffeur, whom Bonney himself had taught to fish. Fishing on the Wye is now greatly restricted, both by natural events causing fewer salmon to rise there and the European Union regulations, which do not allow any fish to be caught before June. George Bonney was a frequent visitor in later years, taking part in the fishing also.

By 1949 (Figure 20), Bonney's operating was very much reduced and he felt his skills were diminishing. Commonly, the visual acuity of a surgeon fades before his manual dexterity. That year he attended a conference on malignant disease in Newcastle where he was fêted. He gave the introductory address on April 1, 1949 and it was later reported in the *Lancet* that Bonney looked back over 30 years of surgical treatment of cervical cancer, giving his final figures as over 500 Wertheim's operations with cure rates of about 40%. He pointed out the uniformity of this result over the long time period, attributing this to his consistency of case selection and surgical techniques. He acknowledged the occasional benefits of adjunct radiotherapy and latterly of pre-operative indication. It must be remembered that this address was given just three years after the dropping of the first atom bombs on Japan. He said: 'Radiotherapy has been the means of greatly increasing our power of destroying life; but alas! not saving it.'

Bonney finished this address, the last major scientific paper he gave, with an elegant compliment to the man he had sparred with for so long in his life, Blair Bell.

'The specific cure for cancer has not yet arrived – some substance or agent which, put into the body, will single out for death the cancer cell, or the factor which energises it, and nothing else. When that day comes, tribute will be paid to Blair Bell, whose work, though it evoked much hostility, largely by reason of his own magnificent egoism, was, I have no doubt of it, along the right path.'

At this time, Bonney turned back to his love of Kipling, feeling that reading his poetry gave him a chance to retreat from the world. It was also at about this time that Bonney stopped even his private operating and so entered full retirement. He was in his late seventies. Bonney felt the position of the United Kingdom had been greatly undermined by two world wars. He knew of the difficulty in getting raw materials to keep heavy industry going efficiently. He considered that the behaviour of the unions was a disadvantage to British industry, and that there was a great spirit of discontent in the country. Materialism was competing with organised religion.

Bonney and Annie attended the London Congress of the Royal College of Obstetricians and Gynaecologists in 1949, staying at Claridges. He was saluted at the Congress as an international pioneer. At a Congress dinner, held by the consultant staff at Chelsea Hospital for Women, he was presented with a gold watch which he greatly treasured. This was inscribed with the words 'In Gratitude'.

In his later retirement Bonney occupied himself reading and listening to the wireless. He would willingly converse with any visitors or friends who called by. He did not often go to London and he did not fish. He was not allowed to garden by Annie who considered that was her empire. He painted marine pictures and the scenery of the area.

The end came fairly swiftly. Having been well until the spring of 1953, Bonney developed a chest infection and was unable to attend a dinner to have been given in his honour. He had a coronary thrombosis whilst at home, diagnosed clinically by his general practitioner. Bonney was transferred by ambulance to a private wing of the Middlesex. There he seemed to be doing well and was visited several times by his family. One of his last visitors was Sir William Gilliatt, then President of the Royal College of Obstetricians and Gynaecologists. Bonney told him that he was 'tired of being in hospital and wanted to get out because he had so much work to do'. Unexpectedly, Bonney had a cerebrovascular accident and fell unconscious. He fortunately did not linger long and died on July 4. Obituaries full of praise were written by many professional and establishment figures, for the man was internationally known as the gynaecological surgeon who founded a dynasty of surgeons. Bonney was buried at Putney Vale Cemetery next to his father.

# CHAPTER ELEVEN

# L'ENVOI
## *1872–1953*

---

*Concerning brave Captains*
*Our age hath made known*
*For all men to honour,*
*One standeth alone*
RUDYARD KIPLING, *GREAT HEART*

B onney lived in the last days of a secure phase in British society. His adult life included the reigns of Victoria, Edward VII, George V and George VI with a working life from about 1905 to 1945. He spent 40 years near or at the apex of a most conservative medical profession. There is no doubt that Bonney was a master surgeon, probably the finest of his class in gynaecology.

It is hard for us at the beginning of the twenty-first century to remember the conditions under which Bonney had to work. Anaesthesia was primitive. Either chloroform or ether was given through an open gauze mask or a closed circuit, which asphyxiated the patient with their own carbon dioxide. Relaxation of the abdominal wall muscles was not performed, and retractors were not in common use. One can only imagine what the conditions were with a tight abdominal wall and no relaxation. The assistants had to hold open the incision with their hands to allow Bonney a limited field for surgery. Blood transfusion was hardly used in the earlier part of his surgical career, its introduction being stimulated by the First World War. Douglas MacLeod, one of his assistants, used to say that it was only in the last hundred of Bonney's 500 Wertheim's operations that blood transfusion played a significant part. The fifth edition of *Ten Teachers* (published in 1935, almost at the end of Bonney's active surgical life) gives only a scant account of how to set up a blood transfusion and 'How to ascertain to which blood group a particular individual belongs'. Cross matching was empirical, and this 1935 edition describes how 'the Red Cross keep a list of persons who have volunteered to be donors'. Sulphonomide treatment of sepsis only began in 1935, becoming widely available after the Second World War. All cases before then had to face the hazards of sepsis. Bonney played his part in reducing this with his Bonney's Blue dye. These and many other practical problems were all hazards the modern surgeon does not need to consider, and yet Bonney moved into a major field of surgery facing them every time he performed a major operation.

It is difficult to designate in any age the greatest person of any field. Even at the summit of Everest there is room for two or three people to stand, and undoubtedly Bonney would be amongst the cluster of the greatest surgeons between the wars. He was not merely a good technical gynaecological surgeon who had learnt his anatomy well in youth; he was also a man of immense resource and observational powers. Further, he was a passionate teacher. Frank Cook, who knew his work well, describes his surgical career:

'Victor Bonney, above all others, created and perfected gynaecological surgery in this country and indeed the whole world. He was a clear and scientific thinker, a superb craftsman and a supreme surgeon. He was intellectually honest and conscientious to a degree. In spite of (or possibly because of) his great experiences and achievements, he was actually a modest man with the humble outlook of the truly great.'

Having been well trained and practised in general surgery, Bonney had no fears about operating on anything he met during gynaecological operations. The bowel, the gallbladder and the urinary tract were all in his domain and on each he would operate electively, as is shown in the operating case analysis in Appendix iii. He particularly pioneered the Wertheim's hysterectomy, performing a great number of these, of which the earlier ones were in combination with Comyns Berkeley. Wertheim himself was quite unpopular, and his operation was in danger of being completely rejected by British surgeons. This may have been because of the nationality of the surgeon or more possibly because it was such a difficult piece of surgery to perform. The advent of radiotherapy has reduced the usage of radical surgical treatments, but it is still extremely useful in younger women with early stages of cancer of the cervix. As well as this, Bonney pioneered conservative gynaecological surgery as seen in his work on ovarian cystectomy and myomectomy. He left his mark on Caesarean section where he was one of the early surgeons to employ the lower segment operation. This was an area of the uterus that some surgeons did not believe existed before labour. They alleged he was operating on something that was not there, but Bonney (with a smile) would continue his work using his own design of haemostatic equipment and achieving excellent results. On one occasion at Chelsea Hospital for Women, he was demonstrating this technique to his consultant colleagues who were an argumentative audience. They tried to throw Bonney, but all failed for he had an indisputable reason for everything he did. Bonney's Test for the assessment of the potential usefulness of repair surgery for anterior vaginal wall prolapse is still used and referred to as such around the world. He was an operative obstetrician interested in the surgical side of the subject, although he always paid attention to the whole woman, and the psychological aspects of patient care concerned him considerably.

Bonney was a great teacher. He started early and while a tutor at the Middlesex Hospital in the first days of the century he supplemented his salary by coaching, tackling all subjects: 'but then I had a wonderful parrot memory'. It was more than the memory, however, that led pupils to beat a path to his door. He was a logical teacher and sets of his tutorial notes were handed down all over the British Empire for years afterwards. In postgraduate teaching at the Middlesex and Chelsea Hospitals, and later at the Hammersmith, he was without peer and inspired devotion, enthusiasm and loyalty in the young men who worked with him. Often towards the end of an operation, between singing snatches from *Tosca*, Bonney would suggest a piece of research arising from the case, which his young assistants would then carry out.

All these abilities arose in a man who was small, sharp and basically reserved. Perhaps those who know about childhood influences would link this with the fact that he had a rather lonely childhood. He did not mix with other children outside the family until the end of his first decade of life, being taught at home by his parents. The society in which he moved as a boy was entirely adult, and he was allowed to join in with the singing concerts and the other social events of the Bonney household. He had a photographic memory and grew up with a logical approach to all new facts, linking them to previous ones he had learned. Despite this, he did not do well in early examinations; he soon realised, however, that a quick flash review of the facts the day before was not enough and he had to do some thinking about the subject as well. This revelation came to him at his time of qualification and, as with so many doctors, his real training took place from then on. Some would say he was stubborn. In debate, Bonney would challenge his consultant colleagues with a point of view that they did not hold. However, he was obdurate for he always knew he was right, and in later years this was often shown to be so.

Bonney would probably have been a good family man, but was denied the opportunity by Annie's early hysterectomy. He made up for this by looking after the members of his extended family. Bonney cared for his brother's children both financially and by offering a fatherly attitude to them. His niece, the daughter of Annie's sister, Irene, lived with the Bonneys for some years and he devoted to her the attention he would have given to a daughter. He had a strong bond to both his private and public patients, and would turn out at any hour of the day or night in order to help them. His habit of calling everybody 'Darling' was surprising at first to some, but it soon became part of the background. One of his assistants commented that, whilst operating, the more endearing Bonney became the worse it boded for everybody. If he changed from 'Darling' to 'Dearest' it was positively dangerous. He was courteous in his relations with the nursing staff and kind to them if he thought they needed his help, but being a shy man he never pressed himself forwards.

He had a busy routine of about 18 hours a day, starting early in the morning, working all day and then enjoying dinner with friends. He would often go on dancing afterwards, a pursuit at which he excelled as a neat, svelte performer with Annie. He enjoyed his comfortable life and as his professional work reduced he spent more time in Hereford. There he was surrounded by his books and paintings, while his friends used to come down to see him. There was a generation of surgeons whom he trained, all of whom were devoted to him; many made the pilgrimage down to Seabournes.

Annie was his lifetime love and companion. She outlived him by a decade, only leaving Seabournes about five years after his death to return to a flat in London. She kept an excellent house and was a constant and caring companion to Bonney. Bonney was devoted to her and she to him. When she left Seabournes it was sold and George Bonney, a nephew, bought one of the cottages on the river, visiting there with his wife for some years.

Bonney's great surgical palaces have mostly crumbled. Chelsea Hospital for Women closed in 1986, moving into the same building as the Queen Charlotte's Hospital for Women in Goldhawk Road. The twin hospitals are in the process of being absorbed into the Hammersmith Hospital where a wing is being built for them. It is to be hoped that Bonney's name will be remembered in some area of the new hospital. The Middlesex Hospital has combined with University College Hospital and the Royal Free Hospital, while the Masonic Hospital has now closed. The Royal College of Surgeons goes from strength to strength advising government, sometimes without much response, about surgical training and surgical standards. The Royal College of Obstetricians and Gynaecologists has flourished from its early days when Bonney was uncertain of its formation and is now accepted by the medical establishment as the source of information about training and standards in the subject. Many of the old traditions that Bonney knew as a surgeon have gone. The Chelsea Hospital Clinical Society once met and dined on the shillings left over from the guineas, but it closed in 1999. The Victor Bonney Society still perpetuates his memory among younger gynaecologists. There is an annual lecture named after him at the RCOG, when a subject, usually in the field of gynaecological malignancy, is dealt with by his second-generation successors.

Bonney was one of the great men of his generation, in an era that has passed on. Perhaps now we rely more on multidisciplinary activities than on the giants of surgery, so many of whom strode the operating theatres of the 1920s. However, as well as his surgical ability, his kindness of heart and the fact that he never failed a colleague or a friend will be remembered. As Gordon Gordon-Taylor, quoting Horace, said in his last words on Bonney:

'INTEGER VITAE SCELERISQUE PURUS'

# SOURCES QUOTED

1.  Bonney V. Then and now. *St Bartholomew Hosp J* September
    1950
    A lecture given to St. Bartholomew's Hospital students at the
    Abernethian Society when Bonney was 77.

2.  The manuscript of a speech prepared by Bonney, to have been
    given at a dinner celebrating his eightieth birthday in 1952.
    Unfortunately he was ill and this speech was never given but it
    remains in the family papers in manuscript form.

3.  Berkeley C, Bonney V. The Middlesex Hospital at Clacton-on-
    Sea during the Great War 1914–1919. *Arch Middlesex Hosp*
    1920;42(Suppl)

4.  Sir Gordon Gordon-Taylor's obituary of Victor Bonney (1953).

5.  Bonney V. The necessity of recognising midwifery as a branch
    of surgery. *Br Med J* 1913;I:552–4

6.  Bonney V. The camps of the southernmost legions. *Middlesex
    Hosp J* 1929;29:41–50,87–94
    An account of Bonney's Australasian visit.

7.  Letters in archives of Royal College of Obstetricians and
    Gynaecologists, 1928–9

# THE CHRONOLOGY OF VICTOR BONNEY'S LIFE

| YEAR | PROFESSIONAL ACTIVITIES | OTHER ACTIVITIES | UK & WORLD EVENTS |
|------|-------------------------|------------------|-------------------|
| 1872 | | Bonney born, December 17 | Gladstone Prime Minister |
| 1890 | Medical School (St. Bartholemew's and Middlesex Hospitals) | | |
| 1893 | | Family moves to 110 Elm Park Gardens | |
| 1895 | Qualifies (Conjoint) | | |
| 1896 | Qualifies (MB) | | |
| 1897 | HP Middlesex     MD | | |
| 1898 | Middlesex Casualty Senior House Officer | | |
| 1899 | Chelsea Hospital for Women – RMO     MS | | Boer War begins (ends 1902) |
| 1900 | Queen Charlotte's Hospital – RMO     FRCS | Engaged to Annie Appleyard | |
| 1901 | Chelsea Hospital for Women – Registrar  MRCP | | Queen Victoria dies Edward VII crowned |
| 1903 | Outpatient gynaecologist at Chelsea Hospital for Women | | Entente Cordiale with France |
| 1904 | Registrar at the Middlesex Hospital Gains a BSc in Anatomy Stops private practice of obstetrics | | |
| 1905 | | Marries Annie Appleyard | |
| 1907 | Middlesex assistant obstetric/gynaecological surgeon Hunterian Professor, RCS | Annie has a hysterectomy | |
| 1908 | His first publication on Wertheim's operation | | |

| YEAR | PROFESSIONAL ACTIVITIES | OTHER ACTIVITIES | UK & WORLD EVENTS |
|---|---|---|---|
| 1909 | Obstetric/gynaecological surgeon, Middlesex Hospital | | |
| 1910 | | | Edward VII dies |
| 1911 | First edition of *Gynaecological Surgery* | | George V crowned National Insurance Act |
| 1912 | Consultancy at Greenwich and Putney Hospitals GVS founded | | |
| 1913 | Full consultant gynaecologist at Chelsea Hospital for Women | | |
| 1914 | Bonney travels to Clacton Hospital three days a week (to 1919) | | First World War begins (ends 1918) |
| 1916 | Bonney's Blue is described | | Gallipoli campaign |
| 1917 | | | Passchendaele battle |
| 1918 | | Bonney's mother dies | Lloyd George's Liberal government is elected |
| 1919 | | | League of Nations is formed |
| 1920 | | Bonney's father dies | |
| 1921 | | | Chelsea Hospital Clinical Society is started |
| 1922 | Bonney's myomectomy clamp described | | |
| 1923 | President of the Obstetric and Gynaecological Section of the RSM | Train visit to Italy | |
| 1926 | Member of Council of RCS | Egypt visit | General Strike |
| 1927 | | Australasia visit | Blair Bell starts BCOG campaign |
| 1929 | Hunterian professor, RCS | | BCOG founded |
| 1930 | | | |
| 1931 | Senior Surgeon in Gynaecology (Middlesex Hospital) | Seabournes bought | UK financial collapse |
| 1933 | Resigns from Chelsea Hospital for Women Bradshaw lecturer, RCS | | |
| 1935 | | USA visit | George V Silver Jubilee |
| 1936 | Vice-president RCS (for three years) | | George V dies Edward VIII abdicates |
| 1937 | Member of Gynaecological Club | | George VI crowned |

| YEAR | PROFESSIONAL ACTIVITIES | OTHER ACTIVITIES | UK & WORLD EVENTS |
|---|---|---|---|
| 1938 | Resigns from Middlesex Hospital | | |
| 1939 | Joins BPMS and Royal Masonic Hospital | | Second World War begins (ends 1945) |
| 1940 | Inspector of Red Cross hospitals (West Country) | | Air raids |
| 1941 | Locum at Cheltenham Hospital (to 1945) | | |
| 1942 | | Penland's bust of Bonney sculpted | V1 raids |
| 1943 | Hunterian oration, RCS | | Royal Charter granted to BCOG |
| 1945 | | | Atomic bombs dropped on Japan |
| 1946 | Leaves Council of RCS Accepts honorary FRCOG | | |
| 1948 | | | NHS introduced |
| 1950 | Congress of RCOG | | |
| 1953 | | Bonney dies, July 4 | |

- *BCOG* – British College of Obstetricians and Gynaecologists
- *BPMS* – British Postgraduate Medical School
- *RCM* – Royal College of Surgeons
- *RCOG* – Royal College of Obstetricians and Gynaecologists
- *RSM* – Royal Society of Medicine

# THE PUBLISHED WORKS
# OF VICTOR BONNEY

The following list is based on Bonney's own curriculum vitae:

## BOOKS

- *A Textbook of Gynaecological Surgery.* Cassell and Co.
  (with Comyns Berkeley)
  1st edition, 1911
  2nd edition, 1919
  3rd edition, 1935
  4th edition, 1942
  5th edition, 1948
  6th edition, 1952

- *The Difficulties and Emergencies of Obstetrics.* London: J & A Churchill.
  (with Comyns Berkeley)
  1st edition, 1913
  2nd edition, 1915
  3rd edition, 1921
  Spanish edition, 1917

- *A Guide to Gynaecology in General Practice.* London: J & A Churchill.
  (with Comyns Berkeley)
  1st edition, 1914
  2nd edition, 1917
  3rd edition, 1920

- *Cancer of the Uterus. Postgraduate Lectures.* Bale, Son and Danielson, 1925.

- *The Technique of Myomectomy.* 1936.

- *The Abnormal in Obstetrics.* London: Edward Arnold, 1938.
  (with Comyns Berkeley and Douglas MacLeod)

- *Extended Myomectomy and Ovarian Cystectomy.* Cassell and Co. Hoeber and Co. (Harpers), 1946.

## CHAPTERS IN BOOKS

- *Eden and Lockyer's New System of Gynaecology.* 1915
- Puerperal sepsis. In *Hutchison's Index of Treatment* (6th edition to 11th edition). 1916–1934.
- Diseases of the female genital tract. In *Walton's Textbook of Surgical Diagnosis.* London: Edward Arnold, 1928.
- The female genital tract. In *Choyce's System of Surgery* (1st edition and 2nd edition). Cassell and Co, 1923 and 1933

- Various chapters in *The Ten Teachers: Midwifery* (1st to 5th edition). London: Edward Arnold, 1917–1938
- Various chapters in *The Ten Teachers: Diseases of Women* (1st to 5th edition). London: Edward Arnold, 1918–1938
- *Encyclopaedia of Midwifery and Diseases of Women.* Fairbairn J, ed. Oxford: Oxford Medical Publications, 1926
- Piersol GM. *The Cyclopaedia of Medicine.* 1934

## ARCHIVES OF THE MIDDLESEX HOSPITAL AND MIDDLESEX HOSPITAL JOURNAL

- Modern views concerning the implantation of the ovum. *Middlesex Hosp J* 1904;8:68–77
- Some aspects of inflammation. *Middlesex Hosp J* 1904;8:10–16
- The cytology of papilliferous ovarian cysts. *Arch Middlesex Hosp* 1904:178–88
- Tubal gestation. A pathological study [with Comyns Berkeley]. *Arch Middlesex Hosp* 1905;4:1–27
- Report of the Obstetrics Register. *Arch Middlesex Hosp* 1905;4:122–132
- On the shortening of labour. *Middlesex Hosp J* 1905;8:251–60
- A new and easy process of triple staining for cytological purposes, founded on Fleming's 'Triple' Stain. *Arch Middlesex Hosp* 1905;6:39–42
- On gametoid types of mitosis in the so-called 'gonorrhoeal wart'. *Arch Middlesex Hosp* 1906;7:20–6
- On chorionepithelioma of congenital origin. *Arch Middlesex Hosp* 1906;7:88–106
- The bearings of pathology on the symptoms of tubal gestation. *Arch Middlesex Hosp* 1906;8:65–78
- Report of the Obstetric Registrar. *Arch Middlesex Hosp* 1905;9:96–9
- A study of the connective tissues in squamous cell carcinoma and certain pathological conditions preceding its onset. *Arch Middlesex Hosp* 1907;10:65–72
- On the simulation of the symptoms of tubal pregnancy by acute ovarian-abscess. *Arch Middlesex Hosp* 1908;12:41–7
- A new and rapid triple stain. *Arch Middlesex Hosp* 1908;12:21–3
- The connective tissues in carcinoma and in certain inflammatory states that precede its onset. *Arch Middlesex Hosp* 1908;14:24–79
- The influence of radio-activity on the division of animal cells. *Arch Middlesex Hosp* 1909;15:147–155
- Two cases of total removal of the vagina, uterus and appendages by para-vaginal section [with Comyns Berkeley]. *Arch Middlesex Hosp* 1909;17:18–28
- A case of utriculoplasty for uterine haemorrhage. *Arch Middlesex Hosp* 1910;18:22
- A case of Caesarean section after attempted delivery by craniotomy. *Arch Middlesex Hosp* 1910;20:23–7
- On post-operative paralytic obstruction of the intestine, with special reference to its treatment by jejunostomy. *Arch Middlesex Hosp* 1910;21:39–48
- Case of double uterus and vagina in which total hysterectomy was performed. *Arch Middlesex Hosp* 1911;24:31–6

- On three cases of acute hepatic intoxication following abdominal section in which jaundice was a marked feature. *Arch Middlesex Hosp* 1912;25:8–13
- A case of rupture of the vagina during coitus. *Arch Middlesex Hosp* 1913;28:57–60
- The results of seventy one examinations of cervical cancer. *Arch Middlesex Hosp* 1913;31:1–6
- The Middlesex Hospital at Clacton-on-Sea during the Geat War (1914–1918). *Arch Middlesex Hosp* 1920;42 (Suppl)
- The paths to the stars. *Middlesex Hosp J* 1927;27:161–7
- The camps of the southernmost legions. *Middlesex Hosp J* 1929;29:41–50,87–94
- Comyns Berkeley, an appreciation. *Middlesex Hosp J* 1931;31:141–56
- Kipling and doctors. *Middlesex Hosp J* 1936;36:41–4

## TRANSACTIONS OF THE ROYAL SOCIETY OF MEDICINE AND PROCEEDINGS OF THE ROYAL SOCIETY OF MEDICINE

- Leukoplakic vulvitis and its relation to kraurosis vulvae and carcinoma vulvae [with Comyns Berkeley]. *Trans R Soc Med* 1909;3:29–51
- Adenomatosis vaginae: a hitherto undescribed condition. (with Bryden Glendinning]. *Trans R Soc Med* 1913;6:121–2
- An ovarian dermoid cyst expelled through the rectum during labour. *Trans R Soc Med* 1914;7:226–7
- Uterus showing squamous-cell carcinoma of the cervix and adeno-carcinoma of the body. *Trans R Soc Med* 1914;7:227–8
- Hernia into the umbilical cord. *Trans R Soc Med* 1914;7:228–9
- On postoperative thrombosois. *Proc R Soc Med* 1928;January 18
- The results of Wertheim's operation and a comparison between them and radium. *Proc R Soc Med* 1929;22:53–68
- Specimen of scar implantation endometrioma. *Proc R Soc Med* 1932;25:69–74
- Frequency of micturition in women. *Proc R Soc Med* 1932;25:1569–71
- Leukoplakic vulvitis and the conditions liable to be confused with it. *Proc R Soc Med* 1935;28:1057–60
- Hydrops foetalis [with H.J.S. Morton]. *Proc R Soc Med* 1938;31:1060–7
- The diagnosis and treatment of acute abdomen from the gynaecological point of view. *Proc R Soc Med* 1943;36:530–1
- Chronic vulval skin lesions [with R.T. Brain]. *Proc R Soc Med* 1944;37:431–3

## JOURNAL OF OBSTETRICS AND GYNAECOLOGY BRITISH EMPIRE AND BRITISH JOURNAL OF OBSTETRICS AND GYNAECOLOGY

- A case of primary infection of the puerperal uterus by Diplococcus pneumonia. *J Obstet Gynaecol Br Emp* 1903;3:177–8
- Intramural rupture of a tubal gestation sac [with Comyns Berkeley]. *J Obstet Gynaecol Br Emp* 1905;7:77–96

- An investigation into the causation of puerperal infections [with A.G.R. Foulerton]. *J Obstet Gynaecol Br Emp* 1905;7:121–6
- On the technique of amputation of the vaginal cervix. *J Obstet Gynaecol Br Emp* 1913;23:121–2
- A case of Caesarean section with remarks on the operation. *J Obstet Gynaecol Br Emp* 1913;24:311–12
- A case of pre-eclampsia at the twenty-fourth week. *J Obstet Gynaecol Br Emp* 1913; 24:313–14
- Results of the radical operation for carcinoma of the cervix uteri. *J Obstet Gynaecol Br Emp* 1913;24:326
- The supporting apparatus of the female genital canal; the displacements that result from the yielding of its several components and the appropriate treatment. *J Obstet Gynaecol Br Emp* 1914;25:328–44
- The modern scope and technique of myomectomy. *J Obstet Gynaecol Br Emp* 1922;29:591–607
- A clamp forceps for controlling haemorrhage when performing myomectomy. *Br J Obstet Gynaecol* 1923;30:447–9
- Diurnal incontinence of urine in women. *J Obstet Gynaecol Br Emp* 1923;30:707–8
- A case in which 52 fibroids were enucleated from the uterus. *J Obstet Gynaecol Br Emp* 1925;32:116–17
- The remoter results of childbearing. *J Obstet Gynaecol Br Emp* 1927;34:419–20
- A further case where endometrial tissue was accidentally implanted. *J Obstet Gynaecol Br Emp* 1928;35:135–6
- The principles that should underlie all operations for prolapse. *J Obstet Gynaecol Br Emp* 1934;41:669–83
- The fruits of conservatism. *J Obstet Gynaecol Br Emp* 1937;44:1–12
- A very large ovarian cyst removed by enucleating it from the ovary (ovarian cystectomy). *J Obstet Gynaecol Br Emp* 1938;45:250–1
- Results of 500 cases of Wertheim's operation for cancer of cervix. *Br J Obstet Gynaecol* 1941;48:421–35
- Division of zygote producing trophoblast only. *Br J Obstet Gynaecol* 1943;50: 217–18
- Unique reconstructive operation [with A.H. McIndoe]. *Br J Obstet Gynaecol* 1944;51:24–9
- Obituary of Sir Comyns Berkeley. *Br J Obstet Gynaecol* 1946;53:109–10
- Surgery of gynaecological surgery. *Br J Obstet Gynaecol* 1947;54:102–6

# LANCET

- The after-treatment and post-operative complicatons of coeliotomy for pelvic disease in women. *Lancet* 1899;ii:337–40
- The treatment of ovarian prolapse by shortening the ovarian ligament. *Lancet* 1906;ii:1726
- Five cases of tumour of the large intestine simulating disease of the uterus or uterine appendages. *Lancet* 1909;ii:525–6
- On occluding and suboccluding ligatures. *Lancet* 1910;ii:455–7
- Six cases of utriculoplasty for uterine haemorrhage. *Lancet* 1911;i:1267–9
- Formation of an artificial vagina by transplantation of a portion of the ileum (Baldwin's operation). *Lancet* 1913;ii:1059–61

- A review of modern gynaecological practice. *Lancet* 1915;ii:1283–9
- On the sole use of Reverdin's needle. *Lancet* 1917;i:994–6
- On abdominal evacuation of the pregnant uterus before viability. *Lancet* 1918;ii:518
- The continued high maternal mortality of childbearing: the reason and the remedy. *Lancet* 1919;i:775–80
- The present position of midwifery. *Lancet* 1920;ii:951–2
- A standardised Reverdin needle and holder. *Lancet* 1921;i:640
- The modern scope and treatment by myomectomy. *Lancet* 1922;ii:745–8
- Gynaecology and general medicine [with H.M. McCrea]. *Lancet* 1923;ii:1025–9
- Abdomino-vaginal excision of the rectum. *Lancet* 1924;i:592–3
- On the inflation test for tubal patency. *Lancet* 1924;ii:1062–3
- The treatment of excessive loss at the periods. *Lancet* 1925;i:938–9
- Injury of the birth canal and the displacements which result from it. *Lancet* 1925; special issue on 'Modern Methods in Abnormal and Difficult Labour'
- Myomectomy as the treatment of election for uterine fibroids. *Lancet* 1925;ii:1060–2
- The major problem of puerperal sepsis. *Lancet* 1926;i:165–89
- The causes and treatment of sterility. *Lancet* 1926;i:865–7
- An operation for creating an abdominal shelf in certain cases of visceroptosis in women. *Lancet* 1926;ii:487–9
- The outcome of 214 radical abdominal operations for carcinoma of the cervix performed five or more years ago. *Lancet* 1926;ii:855
- Malignant disease of the uterus. *Lancet* 1927;ii:31–2,79–80
- On postoperative sepsis in general, and puerperal sepsis in particular. *Lancet* 1928;i:435–8
- Surgical treatment of carcinoma of the cervix. *Lancet* 1930;i:277–82
- The technique and results of myomectomy. *Lancet* 1931;i:171–7
- On sterility. *Lancet* 1932;i:971–5
- Lower segment Caesarean section. The use of Willett's scalp forceps and a uterine compressor. *Lancet* 1933;i:796–7
- The functional derangement of the intestine that follows abdominal operations. *Lancet* 1934;ii:1323–9
- Kipling and doctors. *Lancet* 1937;i:1501–3
- Obituary of Sir John Bland Sutton. *Lancet* 1937;i:50
- Improved uterine dilators. *Lancet* 1939;ii:827
- The forces behind specialism in surgery. *Lancet* 1943;i:669–72
- Wertheim's operation in retrospect. *Lancet* 1949;i:637–9

## BRITISH MEDICAL JOURNAL

- On the radical abdominal operation for carcinoma of the cervix (Wertheim's) [with Comyns Berkeley]. *Br Med J* 1908;II:961–7
- The necessity of recognising midwifery as a branch of surgery. *Br Med J* 1913;I:552–4
- Faecal and intestinal vomiting and jejunostomy. *Br Med J* 1916;I:583–5
- A case of arterio-venous aneurysm of the subclavian artery and vein treated by excision of the sac and the second and third parts of the artery [with

Comyns Berkeley]. *Br Med J* 1916;I:753–5
- The radical abdominal operation for carcinoma of the cervix uteri [with Comyns Berkeley]. *Br Med J* 1916;II:445–7
- Myomectomy or hysterectomy. *Br Med J* 1918;I:278–80
- Sterilisation of the skin and other surfaces by a mixture of crystal violet and brilliant green [with C.H. Browning]. *Br Med J* 1918;I:562–3
- Rabbit-gut. *Br Med J* 1918;II:188
- Proflavine oleate in the treatment of open wounds [with Comyns Berkeley and C.H. Browning]. *Br Med J* 1919;I:152–3
- Pregnancy complicated by volvulus of the pelvic colon. *Br Med J* 1919;II;846
- Obituary notice; Dr. W.A. Bonney [Bonney's father]. *Br Med J* 1920;I:421
- The prevention and treatment of puerperal sepsis. *Br Med J* 1920;II:263–6
- The position of the arms in breech with extended legs. *Br Med J* 1921;I:320
- Remarks on the treatment of acute salpingitis. *Br Med J* 1923;II:400–2
- The surgical treatment of malignant disease of the uterus. *Br Med J* 1925;II:281–4
- Gynaecological considerations in chronic appendicitis. *Br Med J* 1927;II:284
- Path to the stars. *Br Med J* 1927;II:654
- On genital displacements. *Br Med J* 1928;I:431–3
- Australia and New Zealand and our duty thereto. *Br Med J* 1928;II:121–3
- Radium and cancer. *Br Med J* 1928;II:1064
- Operative death rates and professional opinion. *Br Med J* 1930;I:567
- Surgical treatment of carcinoma of the cervix. *Br Med J* 1932;II:307–8
- Results of treatment of cancer of the uterus. *Br Med J* 1934;I:547–9
- Concealed incision of interval appendicectomy. *Br Med J* 1934;II:1005
- Psychological effect of hysterectomy. *Br Med J* 1934;II:1092
- Paralytic ileus after acute appendicitis. *Br Med J* 1935;II:967–8
- Obituary notice: Arthur Giles. *Br Med J* 1936;I:90
- Puerperal sepsis from the point of view of surgery. *Br Med J* 1936;II:342
- Obituary of Blair Bell. *Br Med J* 1936;II:342
- Midwifery in the past and in the present. *Br Med J* 1936;II(Suppl):121–2
- Treatment of carcinoma of the cervix. *Br Med J* 1936;II:1000,1166–7
- Tubo-uterine implantation for sterility. *Br Med J* 1937;I:86
- Corporal punishment. *Br Med J* 1938;I:757–8
- Tetanus bacillus recovered from the scar after ten years [With C. Box and J. MacLennan]. *Br Med J* 1938;II:10–11
- Sterilisation of skin by colourless flavine, 5-amino-acridine [with H.S. Allen]. *Br Med J* 1944;II:210

## OTHER MEDICAL JOURNALS

- Injurious renal mobility ("nephrospasis") in relation to gynaecology. *Edin Med J* 1902;December
- A dermoid cyst containing a large number of epithelial balls. *Trans Obstet Soc* 1902;44:354
- A diphtheroid bacillus isolated from the uterus in two cases of puerperal fever. *Trans Pathol Soc London* 1903;54
- On the homology and morphology of the popliteus muscle. A contribution to comparative myology [with Gordon Gordon-Taylor]. *J Anat Physiol* 1905;40

- The relation between certain physical signs and symptoms in moveable kidney in women. 1905;October 18
- Eine Neue und leicht suszufiihrende dreifache Farbung fiir Zellen und Gewebsschnitte nach Flemmings Dreifachbehandlung. *Virchow's Arch* 1906;185
- On chorionepithelioma of congenital origin. *Trans Pathol Soc London* 1907;548
- Traitement du prolapsus de l'ovaire par le accourcissement du ligament utero-ovarien. *Revu Obstetriq Gynaecologie* 1907
- Eine Neue und Sehr Schnelle Dreifach-Furbung. *Virchow's Arch* 1908;193
- On Puerperal Fever. *Clin J* 1908;32
- Some useful prescriptions in the practice of gynaecology. *Clin J* 1909;34
- The bearings of pathology on the prevention, diagnosis and surgical treatment of carcinoma of the cervix. *Practitioner* 1909;June
- The diagnosis and treatment of haemorrhage from an unenlarged uterus. *Practitioner* 1910;86
- Abdomino-pelvic pain in women without physical signs of disease. *Practitioner* 1911;87
- The diagnosis and operative treatment of carcinoma of the vulva, vagina and uterus. *Practitioner* 1912;88
- Myomectomy as opposed to hysterectomy. *Clin J* 1923;51
- Conservatism in gynaecological surgery. *Practitioner* 1924;March
- The symptoms produced by uterine and vaginal displacements. *Clin J* 1924;53
- The causes and modern treatment of sterility. *Clin J* 1926;55
- The remoter results of childbearing. *Newcastle Med J* 1926
- Conservation of function in gynaecology. *Med J Aust* 1928;June 16
- The making of a surgeon. *J Coll Surg Aust* 1928;July:1
- Urology in relation to gynaecology. *Br J Urol* 1929;March:1
- The diagnosis and treatment of carcinoma of the uterus. *Practitioner* 1931;June
- The technique of Wertheim's operation. *Aust N Z J Surg* 1931;June
- The diagnosis and treatment of fibroids. *Practitioner* 1937;138
- Conservative gynaecological surgery. *S Afr Med J* 1938;February 26
- Merciful and unmerciful surgery. *Med Press* 1941;205:457
- On cancer of the cervix. *Med Press* 1943;209:120
- Treatment of carcinoma of the cervix by Wertheim's operation. *Am J Obstet Gynecol* 1935;30:815
- Functional intestinal obstruction without obvious antecedent cause. *Br J Surg* 1952;40:78

# AN ANALYSIS OF VICTOR BONNEY'S SURGERY AT CHELSEA HOSPITAL FOR WOMEN

### Note on Data from Bonney's Operating Records

Chelsea Hospital for Women closed in 1986. Until that time, clinical records had been stored under each consultant's name and bound together at the end of the year. After temporarily lodging at Queen Charlotte's Hospital, the records were transferred to the London Metropolitan Archives where they are stored in excellent surroundings. Permission to examine the records of Bonney's work was given by the Chief Executive of the Special Trust to whom I am grateful.

At the Archives are 25 volumes of Bonney's hospital notes, some of the books being eight inches thick. The bulk of paper to be examined forced me to examine samples only and so I selected six years at intervals from 1907 to 1934. Inside these sampling limits I read the clinical records of almost 1000 women, but made no copy of the clinical conditions. I recorded the types of operation done by Bonney himself, as judged by the name entered with the procedure (often written in Bonney's own hand).

Scrutiny shows the wide spectrum of surgery Bonney performed. While this was mostly in the pelvis, he was also operating on other areas, e.g. the breast (in the sample years he performed 14 radical mastectomies). His career interests are reflected in the operations he undertook, and it can be seen that conservative operations (myomectomy and ovarian cystectomy) predominated latterly.

Bonney did his operating in two public hospitals: Chelsea Hospital for Women and the Middlesex Hospital. He also operated in a series of private hospitals and homes. This record is a measure of his personal surgery of only one of these places.

**Data overleaf.**

| | 1907 | 1915 | 1919 | 1923 | 1927 | 1930 |
|---|---|---|---|---|---|---|
| Wertheim's hysterectomy | 0 | 9 | 9 | 8 | 4 | 7 |
| Total abdominal hysterectomy | 3 | 7 | 3 | 9 | 14 | 12 |
| Subtotal abdominal hysterectomy | 4 | 19 | 15 | 13 | 37 | 31 |
| Vaginal hysterectomy | 0 | 0 | 0 | 0 | 1 | 1 |
| Myomectomy | 0 | 4 | 6 | 10 | 12 | 18 |
| Ovarian cystectomy or oophorectomy | 3 | 9 | 3 | 10 | 11 | 10 |
| Appendectomy | 0 | 5 | 5 | 5 | 7 | 8 |
| Ventrosuspension | 1 | 14 | 20 | 20 | 38 | 9 |
| Hernia repair | 0 | 4 | 1 | 1 | 5 | 5 |
| Amputation of cervix | 2 | 5 | 22 | 16 | 25 | 6 |
| Anterior repair | 0 | 5 | 3 | 0 | 18 | 19 |
| Posterior repair | 0 | 6 | 20 | 17 | 36 | 14 |
| Examination under anaesthesia | 0 | 6 | 1 | 2 | 4 | 3 |
| Dilatation and curettage of the uterus | 2 | 11 | 11 | 7 | 36 | 35 |
| Marsupialisation of Bartolm's gland | 0 | 2 | 0 | 1 | 0 | 3 |
| Salpingectomy | 0 | 0 | 0 | 4 | 0 | 0 |
| Tubal insufflation | 0 | 0 | 0 | 1 | 13 | 2 |
| Ectopic pregnancy removal | 3 | 1 | 0 | 1 | 0 | 0 |
| Evacuation of pregnancy (termination) | 0 | 0 | 0 | 1 | 0 | 0 |
| Hydatidiform mole | 0 | 0 | 0 | 1 | 0 | 0 |
| Hysterotomy | 0 | 0 | 1 | 2 | 0 | 0 |
| Caesarean section | 1 | 1 | 0 | 1 | 2 | 0 |
| Nephrectomy | 0 | 1 | 0 | 0 | 0 | 0 |
| Cholecystectomy | 0 | 0 | 1 | 1 | 4 | 2 |
| Haemorrhoidectomy | 0 | 0 | 1 | 1 | 0 | 0 |
| Renal stone removal | 0 | 1 | 2 | 1 | 0 | 0 |
| Laparotomy | 0 | 1 | 1 | 0 | 0 | 0 |
| Removal of breast lump | 0 | 2 | 0 | 1 | 5 | 3 |
| Radical mastectomy | 0 | 4 | 3 | 1 | 1 | 5 |
| Plastic enlargement of the introitus | 0 | 0 | 5 | 0 | 1 | 1 |
| Radical excision of rectum | 0 | 1 | 0 | 0 | 0 | 0 |
| Varicose veins resection | 0 | 0 | 5 | 0 | 0 | 0 |
| Pyosalpinx drainage | 1 | 0 | 0 | 0 | 0 | 2 |
| Renal fixation | 0 | 4 | 2 | 1 | 0 | 0 |
| Vulvectomy | 0 | 1 | 0 | 0 | 1 | 3 |
| Reimplantation of tubes | 0 | 0 | 0 | 0 | 1 | 2 |
| Sterilisation | 0 | 0 | 0 | 0 | 2 | 1 |
| Le Fort's repair | 0 | 0 | 0 | 0 | 4 | 1 |
| Vesicovaginal fistula | 0 | 0 | 0 | 0 | 1 | 3 |
| Radium placement | 0 | 0 | 0 | 0 | 0 | 7 |
| Inoperable cancer | 5 | 5 | 0 | 0 | 4 | 6 |
| Other | 1 | 8 | 7 | 4 | 8 | 1 |
| Total | 26 | 136 | 147 | 140 | 295 | 220 |

# THE CHILDHOOD HOMES OF VICTOR BONNEY

| | |
|---|---|
| 1872 | 320 King's Road |
| 1873 | 145 Upper Beaufort Street (West Fulham Road) |
| 1893 | 110 Elm Park Gardens (East Side) |

# THE LONDON CONSULTING ROOMS OF VICTOR BONNEY

| | |
|---|---|
| 1901 | 10 Devonshire Street |
| 1912 | 29 Devonshire Place |
| 1920 | 15 Devonshire Place |
| 1935 | 149 Harley Street (London Clinic) |

# INDEX

**A**

ABC (Aerated Bread Company) 3, 7
Aird, John 96
Alexander, Earl of Athlone 63
Alice, Countess of Athlone (Princess) 63
American Gynaecological Society 92, 102
Appleyard, AC 25–26
Appleyard, Irene 118
Attlee, Clement 105, 109
Aveling, James 15

**B**

Bacon, Miss 19
Baggaley, Mr 5
Baldwin, RW 32–3
Bannister, Bright 31
Barnes, Robert 15
Barrett, Lady 71
Beatty, DB (Admiral) 42
Bedford, Evan 96–97
Bell, William Blair 30, 69, 70, 78, 80, 81,
  83, 85–86, 112
Berkeley, Comyns 17, 20, 24–29, 36–7, 40,
  44, 49, 58–59, 62, 64, 75, 78, 81, 84,
  89–92, 101–102, 105–6, 116
Bevan, Aneurin 107
Bevin, Ernest 105
Blakeley, John 108–109
Boer War 18–20
Bonney, Ernest Henry 1, 25, 91, 93, 96–97
Bonney, Francis 2
Bonney, George 51, 91, 93, 97, 111, 118
Bonney, Gertrude 97
Bonney, Jack 1, 25, 93
Bonney, née Appleyard, Annie 18–20,
  25–27, 29, 35, 41, 50–51, 64–65,
  69–72, 74, 92, 97, 106, 109–112, 118
Bonney, née Poulain, Anna-Maria 1, 5, 45,
  53–54
Bonney, Reginald 74, 92
Bonney, Veronica 97
Bonney, Victor
  and billiards 4–5, 9, 101

and Bonney's Blue 43–44, 106
and Comyns Berkeley's retirement 89–90
and death of Rudyard Kipling 94
and his sympathetic views for his patients
  32–33, 46, 118
and limitation of surgical infection 21,
  47, 106
and membership of RAC club 89
and military service 36–38, 49
and socialising 4, 23, 50–51, 110
and views on midwifery 32, 46
and views on obstetrics as being part of
  surgery 32
and views on politics 47, 52, 77, 90–91,
  94, 96, 99, 105, 109, 112
artistic skill 5, 21–22, 27–28
as a Mason 92
as Inspector of Red Cross Hospitals
  99–101
as locum general practitioner 12
at Seabournes 90, 93, 99–102, 106,
  109–111, 118
Bonney's Test 117
death 113
examinations taken 11–12, 18–19, 21
fishing 26, 30, 50–51, 75–76, 90, 101,
  111
honours and awards 27
love of opera 9, 11, 26
marriage to Annie 25
private practice 19–20, 22, 26, 29–30, 44,
  46, 49, 73, 89, 93, 97, 112
septicaemia 18
surgical technique 31, 69, 73, 77, 92,
  100, 107, 115–117
the smoker 21, 108–109
travels abroad 52, 69
  Egypt 71–72
  New Zealand and Australia 73–76
  USA 92–93
Bonney, William 1–2, 4, 9, 18, 50, 53
Bourne, Alec 69
Boxal, Robert 8

137